Anne Hooper, as a sex therapist, spends much of her time helping couples to re-make contact, sometimes when they haven't touched for years. Anne Hooper, as a journalist and author, tries to clarify, in writing, the important link between feeling happy and being close to other human beings. Anne Hooper, as a phone-in counsellor for LBC Radio, helps people with problems find new options for themselves which may include using touch to show they care. Anne Hooper, as a partner and mum, cuddles her long-suffering family at the slightest opportunity.

As well as writing for a number of magazines, Anne Hooper is the author of *Divorce and Your Children* (Unwin Paperback), *The Body Electric* (Unwin Paperback) and *Women and Sex* (Sheldan Press). She has three children and lives in London.

D0317115

Massage and Loving

Massage and Loving

ANNE HOOPER

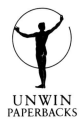

UNWIN
PAPERBACKS

LONDON SYDNEY WELLINGTON

First published in Great Britain by Unwin ® Paperbacks, an imprint
of Unwin Hyman Limited in 1988

UNWIN HYMAN LIMITED
15/17 Broadwick Street
London W1V 1FP

Allen & Unwin Australia Pty Ltd
8 Napier Street, North Sydney, NSW 2060, Australia

Allen & Unwin New Zealand Pty Ltd with Port Nicholson Press
60 Cambridge Terrace, Wellington, New Zealand

Hooper, Anne
  Massage and loving.
  I. Sex relations. Role of massage
  I. Title
613.9′6

ISBN 0–04–613068–3

Typeset by Cambrian Typesetters, Frimley, Surrey
and Printed in Great Britain at
The University Press, Cambridge

Photographs by Charles Roff
Photograph page 81 Ian Sanderson
Illustrations by Alicia Durdos
Designed by Julia Lilauwala

To Phillip

Contents

Contents

Introduction

The way we touch people makes an impression from the moment we meet. If we touch with warmth and assurance we invite warmth and appreciation in return. If we caress sensually, we provoke sensuality. With lovers, touch is the most immediate and important means of demonstrating love and providing reassurance.

Yet touch does not come spontaneously to everyone. Our sensual backgrounds, the way we were brought up, whether or not our parents provided an example of love and affection, have a direct impact on our ability to express ourselves physically.

All the same we can *learn* to be demonstrative and to enhance our own powers of attraction by discovering how to touch. Cuddling, hugging, caressing, these are the first experiences any of us enjoy and it is on these early experiences that we build our later confidence and sexuality. The cuddling we receive as babies actually builds pathways and networks in the brain assembling a cerebral apparatus for the recognition and enjoyment of sensation. If we don't get the caresses, the brain fails to construct these particular channels and we grow up intrinsically different from other human beings.

Dr James Prescott, an American neuro-psychologist, claims that the absence or withdrawal of physical affection in early life and even as an adult may be responsible for many types of disturbed behaviour such as depression, sexual inhibition, drug abuse, violence, aggression and hyperactivity. He has produced enough evidence to make scientists take his ideas seriously. Experiments with animals show that when the parts of their brains known to produce pleasure are stimulated, their aggressiveness diminishes. And when the animals are given regular physical affection, they behave with increased stability.

Dr Prescott's work with primitive societies shows that people who are physically affectionate towards their children generally live in non-violent cultures, whereas people who are physically cold and forbidding towards adolescents produce aggressive, hostile and sometimes violent offspring.

To this Dr Prescott adds his view that the positive benefits of warm, affectionate touching during childhood may sometimes be undone by sensual repression in teenage. Equally, the absence of sensory pleasure during infancy can also be mitigated provided there is a permitted degree of sensual pleasure during adolescence. In St Albans' Hill End Hospital, England, disturbed teenagers go through an intensive course of physical treatment, learning to appreciate the significance of touching and being touched. Since this kind of therapy has been introduced violence at the hospital has noticeably abated.

If we use the fundamental principles of nurturing when beginning a new relationship, it helps create an atmosphere of trust. When someone caresses or massages your body your ego feels stroked too. This is a form of love. Doing the same to others is equally good therapy since giving your partner pleasure brings you pleasure.

Touch can be used in infinite ways. Thus a massage can eliminate aggression, a cuddle can heal a quarrel, holding someone close helps deal with feelings of grief. Embracing a friend while you give bad news cushions the impact, stroking, patting and hugging your spouse, your children *and* your friends can let them know how much you care for them.

A television documentary made some years ago about touching showed that shoppers remembered the shop assistant better if she briefly touched them when she proffered their change. Research on job interviews shows that interviewers receive a more favourable impression of the applicant who shakes their hand than the one who does not. American research indicates that patients touched by nurses were reassured, their anxiety reduced and they calmed down. Even patients in a coma registered a significant response when a nurse routinely took their pulse.

Dr Prescott's theory, that a dose of sensuality in later life can socialise and introduce people to pleasure they should have known in earlier life, is one of the few good arguments in favour of sexual surrogates. On the west coast of America, hot tubs are used in fringe maritial therapy, manipulation is taught to heighten communication between young marrieds, and 'growth weekends', which include bodywork, foster feelings of well-being and happiness.

Massage is a deliberate and concentrated form of touch. In the past it has been used for remedial purposes and as an adjunct to athletic performance. Historically, massage has been central to the more body-conscious civilisations, such as classical Rome, where an entire way of life was virtually designed around the thermal bath.

Here in the UK and the US we have partly lost touch with the pleasures and benefits of such a physical lifestyle. Perhaps our climate has clouded our body-consciousness; perhaps we have handed down a national inhibition about nudity. Whatever the reason our main contribution to massage to date has been an unacceptable one – the phoney massage parlour.

Although genital release parlours may have their place, the 'sauna-sex' business has damaged the cause of massage. Yet the ancient skills have a knack of springing back in modern times. Bio-feedback machines, products of this electronic age, show how to control anxiety and stress by measuring electrical impulses in our skin. A vital part of the bio-feedback therapy consists (besides meditation) of *healing touch*.

All recent attempts to formulate sex therapy are founded on laboratory analysis of human sexual response. Electrodes and mechanical equipment have explained what happens physiologically when we make love. Yet the practical curative work is carried out through deliberate touching exercises called 'sensate focus', or *mutual massage* by any other name.

Even the verbal method of present-day analysis has a 'body-version' in rolfing. Rolfing is a form of *aggressive massage* that works deep into the body 'armour' formed by knotted muscles and iron-clad body tension. Through softening up this 'armour' clients are able to become less rigid in releasing emotional attitudes and behaviour.

So far modern massage has been reserved either for those desperate enough to enter the massage parlour or those daring enough to seek the selective therapeutic help described. That leaves millions of us who fit into neither of these two categories – people who could use massage every day in personal relationships if only we knew how to go about it.

By doing so we could simply improve our lives and give them a sensual tang. Or tan. Just as most of us feel a flow of happiness when we bare our bodies to the summer sun so could we feel that same glow when we bare our limbs to the pressures of caring fingers. Touch doesn't only mean sensation, it also means an emotional caring experience. This is what makes touch a foundation for love.

Massage can be used at every major part of the life cycle so that it seems as natural as holding hands or linking arms. And this can be done matter-of-factly enough for all hints of trendiness to vanish. The intention of this book, therefore, is to show how all of this is possible. I want to demonstrate ways in which you can give pleasure to your friends and family and feel absolutely fine about doing it.

The book isn't designed to be a dictionary, but it is written so that the connection between beginning a touch lesson and beginning a new friendship is made clear. Indeed, the analogies are there all through the life cycle. Marriage, for example, is a type of continuity and again a link is made in these pages between learning continuity of touch and continuing to work at a married relationship.

On the following pages are soothing strokes to take tension out of life for friends, sensual strokes to turn lovers on, simple touch games two people can play to make life fun, touch to show a child you care – enough in fact to last for a lifetime of touch.

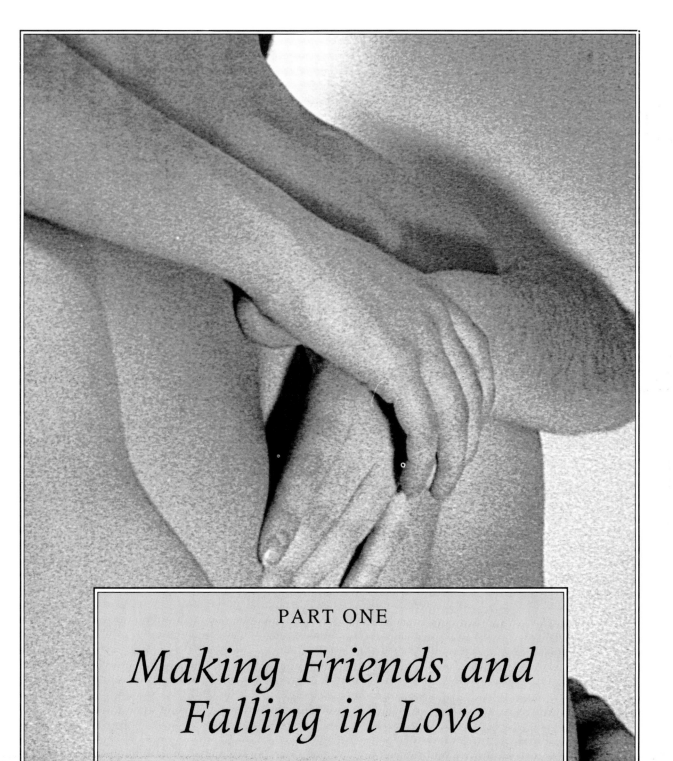

PART ONE

Making Friends and Falling in Love

Growing comfortable with touch – beginnings

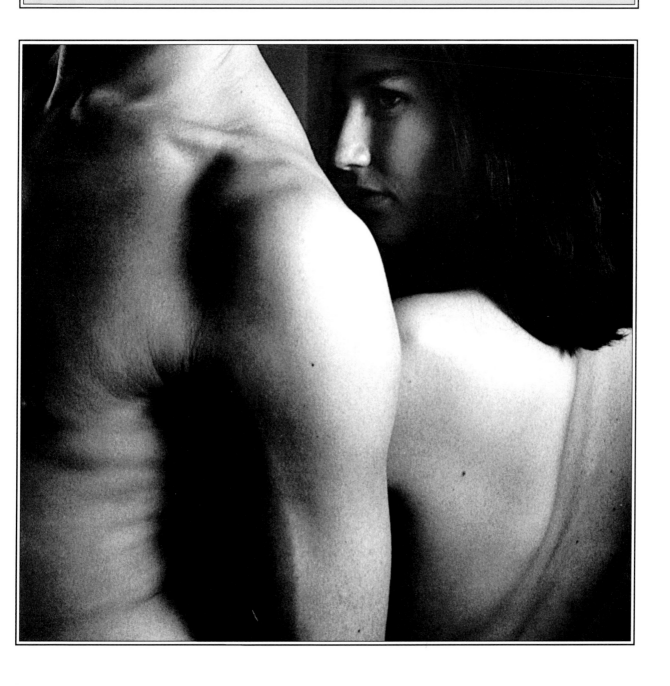

Reassurance through touch

The first sensation that means anything to us is touch. Floating in our mother's womb, the soft swirling of water around our tiny body will have created sensations. It is from these sensations that we build our very earliest awarenesses. Small wonder then that something as basic as 'skin nourishment' – in other words, stroking, caressing, hugging – gives us a feeling of well-being. But it does more than just make us feel good. It is actually responsible for our will to live.

There is some now famous research, carried out fifty years ago by Dr Rene Spitz of the New York Foundling Hospital, which revealed a fascinating insight. Although the babies in the Foundling Hospital were kept well fed and in clean conditions, they had a high death rate. Holidaying in Mexico Dr Spitz observed babies in a local orphanage, not so clean and well fed, but nevertheless happier and healthier than those in in the Foundling Hospital. The difference lay in the fact that the village women came into the orphanage every day and played with the children. They fondled, stroked and talked to the babies, while, in New York, the children were left strictly alone in their cradles. Dr Spitz's observations led to a famous study which confirmed that the stimulation of touch was vital to life.

Many of us were touched frequently by our parents during such occasions as nappy-changing, bathtime and simply through being carried, when we were tiny. But as we left infancy and grew older, the touching sadly grew less. Older children often have to survive without loving touch at all. Certainly most children withdraw from parental touch during adolescence.

Think for a moment of the comfort that maternal touching brings. Have you ever noticed the first thing a mother does when her toddlers falls over? She picks him up and gives him a good cuddle. It is her warm skin sensations which help calm him down. Physiologically her embrace triggers off certain chemicals inside the child which are discharged into his bloodstream and which are responsible for altering his mood and cheering him up.

One of the first things lovers do after making up a quarrel is to embrace, each seeking reassurance from their loving intimacy. They are following a similar pattern. When someone has had a shock it is common to comfort them by holding them close.

Comfort apart, touch gives simple encouragement. If we *don't* get bodily gratification from our parents, theorises neuro-psychologist Dr James Prescott, we can grow up to be violent and delinquent. Certainly the famous monkey research by Harry Harlow in the late 1950s bears this out. Monkeys which received inadequate mothering were fierce, aggressive, even violent.

The teens are a period of acute self-consciousness – an awareness brought on by the escalation of skin sensation. As sex hormones flood the system, thanks to the onset of puberty, they bring, among other things, greatly enhanced skin sensitivity. We realise, as never before, the sensuality of touch. The skin tingles in a new way; areas of the body grow receptive to touch which previously felt little; sensual circuits rush into overload; young men get erections at a glance; young women develop passions and flirtations. Bathing in front of parents becomes taboo for the first time. Sexual discussion between parent and child which was acceptable at the age of 12 is cut right out of the conversation at the age of 13. Brushing against a member of the opposite sex is fraught with accidental arousal.

As a result of this new sensuality young people no longer allow themselves to touch with the spontaneity of childhood. They withdraw, reserving touch very specifically for someone trustworthy, such as a first lover. Indeed, one of the reasons we need first lovers, not to mention subsequent ones, is *because* we have withdrawn from our parents and are suffering from skin starvation. (The need to be touched can be extreme enough to prompt sexual overtures in the face of the most blatant rejection. It was the need to be touched, says one survey of twenty women who had had three or more unwanted pregnancies, that led them into sex in the first place.) This touch withdrawal is one which lasts for the rest of our lives, except with specifically chosen lovers and with our own children.

It is at this stage in life, therefore, when we start wanting to make new intimate relationships that we particularly need touch to give us a type of internal balance. With adequate skin attention to nurture us we are likely to be more rational when falling in love, to tread more carefully when making friends and to possess a sense of well-being which is attractive to others.

Setting out to deliberately cultivate a lifestyle which includes maximum touch is the goal which many people have already chosen. But there are many more of us who would like to copy their choice. The dilemma is how to throw ourselves in at the deep end by daring to do something as deliberate as regular massage exercise. Many of us have the will to become more 'physical' with friends, but where (and how) to start? A study of people 'licensed to touch' gives some important clues.

'Licensed' to touch

English and Americans touch each other notoriously less than their European counterparts. (An American survey showed that American friends touch two or three times an hour while European friends touched on average 100 times an hour. The English can expect to be nearer the American score than the European one.) Yet in English/American cultures there are a few situations where touch *is* socially acceptable. People 'licensed' to touch are, for example, doctors, nurses, sports trainers. All have to overcome original inhibitions in order to grow comfortable with touch. The fact they manage to do so indicates touch is not only a matter of hand upon flesh but also *a state of mind.*

Regarding touch as an integral part of a job, therefore, is one way of overcoming inhibition. Overt touch is adapted to become part of a social role and as such becomes socially acceptable. Health students are provided with a host of support and instruction to allow them to do this. They are given, for example, clear rules within their professions about what is and isn't permissible. The mere existence of such rules not only allows them to feel comfortable about touch, but also allows them to transmit their feelings of comfort to others.

While *we* do not have the justification of using touch (and especially massage) in a career, we can find other ways of 'internalising' the belief that touch can be socially acceptable. One way of doing this is *to project an ideal on to yourself.* The image, for example, of a sensitive human being with the power to comfort and heal at the fingertips is a powerful one. Fastening on to that can be the basis for believing that (as far as you and your friends are concerned) massage exercise is a very good idea and even you can become a healer. But to make the links between a 'licensed toucher' and a humble beginner, we need to take a closer look at the route a 'professional' toucher takes. The progress of Peter Hollis, a physiotherapy student, as he grew to feel comfortable with touch is a useful illustration of how someone, unsure of themselves at the commencement of a career internalises feelings of confidence. Once he had achieved this, Peter was able to project his confidence towards his clients so that massage sessions with them were comfortable and relaxed.

Setting up a touch routine

At training college Peter found himself pitchforked into large classes where, amongst other things, he had to learn therapeutic massage. He found the experience of working with so many people in the near nude a hard one in which to feel relaxed. At the suggestion of his teacher, therefore, he advertised within his college for partners on whom he might practise in rather more privacy.

Peter learned that the way to reassure volunteers was to be businesslike from the start. At the initial meeting or telephone discussion he stated how long the massage would last, which parts of the body would receive attention, that at no time would he attempt to be sexually intimate and that if they wanted to bring along a chaperone that would be fine. By doing this, he also reassured himself. The volunteers quickly relaxed within this 'framework' and few of them bothered to bring along a friend to 'supervise'. Peter also explained that he was learning physiotherapy and therefore asked for their patience. He got it.

During his three years as a student Peter shared a flat with several other students who were *not* studying physiotherapy. One of these arrived back from a weekend of fierce rugby with a very stiff leg. Peter offered to massage it. The massage was accepted as it had been given – a straightforward gift to relieve physical discomfort. The other flatmates caught on and Peter discovered he was in demand for anything from a sore knee to a migraine suffered by a grieving friend whose girl had thrown him over. As Peter and his flatmates grew comfortable with Peter's skills, so too did other students. Acquaintances, hearing of Peter's ability to smooth out aches and pains, presented themselves out of the blue. His fame spread. By the end of his studies Peter felt at home with the idea of being a masseur.

When he made the transition from college to city, he chose to move to an area where many of his friends were gathered and where, with a little advertising, he was able to build up a professional clientele. Today Peter is a self-employed physiotherapist who specialises in athletic massage and in aiding men and women with sports injuries.

A detailed examination of Peter's progress reveals a network of moves which could be emulated by anyone. He started off with an advantage – that of studying a 'physical' profession – but where Peter's institute provided him with training and support, this book aims to do the same for the benefit of less formal 'students'.

Peter was helped to find his partners through the existence of his college and through other like-minded fellow students. But a college is only an educational form of 'system' and nearly all of us function within systems of some kind. The family is a system, school another, youth clubs, the area in which we live, marriage and then our own family – all are types of systems which can provide us with 'volunteers'.

Establishing trust

Most people demure at the idea of being 'intimate' with friends. Yet friends and relations are the obvious people to approach first. Peter's example demonstrates how this can be done without a hint of anything sexual. He managed it by establishing himself as someone who could make a friend feel physically better. At the same time he established himself as someone trustworthy who could be relied on not to go too embarrassingly far. He did this by setting up 'rules' within himself. These were: he didn't look for anything other than a head, foot or hand massage to begin with; when he massaged women he didn't 'jump' on them halfway through the massage; he always established trust by: (1) suggesting his volunteers should bring a chaperone and (2) explaining what he was aiming at with each massage. He was open, both with himself and with his friends/ volunteers.

Trustworthiness is a definable quality. Peter's friends describe him by saying that the minute you meet him you sense he is a man to *be* trusted. He projects a feeling of trustworthiness. He learned how to do so. So can we.

The 'inner' process

Peter's example shows us that we need to 'think right' before we can be accepted as 'layers on of hands'. Good touch is an 'inner' process as well as an external one. Part of the inner process rests in being clear about what you expect from your touching. If you have ever experienced a massage from the hands of someone who *expects* a sexual turn-on from your reactions, you will understand the distinction between a 'sexual' massage and a 'sensual' one. A 'sexual' massage acquires an inappropriate tension and a masseur/se who is after a 'sexual reward' won't be someone with whom you will seek a second massage for its own sake. A good masseur does not *expect* a massage to lead up to intercourse or masturbation.

This doesn't mean to say that a massage with a good masseur can't be a wonderfully sensual experience. There is nothing wrong with feeling deliriously sensual, either as massager or as massagee. Nor should you go into a massage attempting to block off all feelings of sensual excitement. But if you expect a sexual ending, or a sexual reward, the quality of the massage is unfavourably altered.

Where to start

There are many of us who find even the thought of massaging difficult! Just how do you get started if you are acutely self-conscious? How do you find that volunteer?

You could do worse than follow Peter's example and offer to smooth away a friend's headache, or to relieve their leg cramps by massaging their calves. *Using occasions which arise spontaneously is one way of beginning.* Peter's other method of raising volunteers was to *advertise* and this can be copied too, if only within your own particular system. Getting the endorsement of an older person or a senior might help. My friend Margaret, while still at school, used to massage her friends in the cloakroom, during the break periods. She was greatly in demand at examination time. It didn't matter that she knew little about massage to start with, she just did 'what came naturally'. Because she was open about it, even practising on the gym teacher, there was never a hint that her activities were 'not quite nice'.

You can encourage friends to volunteer by saying you would like to practise on their head or their hands. The presence of others at a massage may help them feel safe. (One of the reasons Margaret's volunteers felt comfortable was that she was always surrounded by clamorous schoolgirls, fascinated by what she was doing. Cloakrooms are very public places! She couldn't have been 'underhand' if she'd tried.) But the suggestion of a chaperone is a more formal safeguard, calculated to win over the reluctant. And if you are self-conscious, a head massage really lets you off the hook since there isn't apparently a hint of anything sexual about it.

First touches

The mental beginnings of a touch exercise are often ignored. Ray Stubbs, a massage therapist and teacher from San Francisco, prepares himself just before touching by doing something called *centering*. He holds the palms of his hands, an inch or so above his client for a couple of minutes, near enough to feel their warmth without actually resting on their skin. While he does this Ray closes his eyes and imagines that he is breathing in the friend's warmth through his fingertips. This enables him to get a 'feel' of the client before gently lowering his hands on to their skin and beginning the massage – a sort of psychic assessment. One of the advantages to beginners of doing this is that the exercise takes your mind off feeling nervous. There isn't time to feel uncertain when you are experimenting with thermal telepathy!

Ray teaches his students to make hand movements away from the backbone, so that the spine is relieved of stress. He doesn't recommend a lot of specific strokes to begin with, but suggests that a good beginning movement is a *circling* stroke, on the grounds that *any* movement, carried out rhythmically, feels good, and circling is easy to do. In a head and neck massage, therefore, this would mean circling with the thumbs, away from the central part of the neck.

Circling consists of what it sounds like – small circling patterns made with either the thumbs or fingers, or palms and fingers. Ray's other main recommendation is that you should always slow down a massage. It may seem appallingly long and drawn out, at first, but good touch, *done slowly*, is, quite simply, the best.

Spending time, circling the contours of your friends's head, with their eyes closed, is a good start. Ask the friend for feedback. Is your stroke too light or too heavy? Would they prefer lighter pressure or deeper pressure? Ask them to indicate what they really enjoy even if only by the sound of their pleased moans. The more simple practice you put into finding out what is and isn't successful the more confident you will grow.

A positive fact about massage is that it is very pleasurable for the person doing it. Hands are among the body's most touch sensitive areas and massage gives the masseur/se sensual feelings of their own.

Perhaps the most reassuring fact for the very unconfident is that the more massage you do, the better you are likely to feel about doing it. *Touching others is a way of learning to feel better about yourself.*

Non-sexual beginnings

The desirability of establishing trust, of becoming trustworthy, of giving and getting feedback, of *not* rushing the sexual side to a partnership, have their obvious parallels in making relationships *outside* massage. A good relationship benefits from all of these and if you are ambitious to make good friendships, you might do worse than learn how to do so through massage exercise.

Non-sexual beginnings might include putting an arm around a friend, hugging briefly, holding hands, all tentative activities which establish both contact and the degree to which that contact is acceptable. Touch exercise equivalents of these beginning stages are a head massage, a hair massage, a foot massage and an exercise of manipulation and trust. Practising with friends builds up feelings of affection – not to mention giving a lot of fun. At the very least, the following exercises provide grounding for harmony.

The harmonious head – a head massage

One of the secrets of both turning people on and allowing them to enjoy a massage is getting them to relax. So the early harmonious head strokes concentrate on the 'third eye', the energy centre on the forehead above the nose and the gap between the eyebrows. Once tension dissolves here, you experience a wonderful feeling of tranquillity and well-being.

Harmonious Head *Sweep the flat of one hand firmly up and off the forehead, away from the eyes, rapidly followed by the other.*

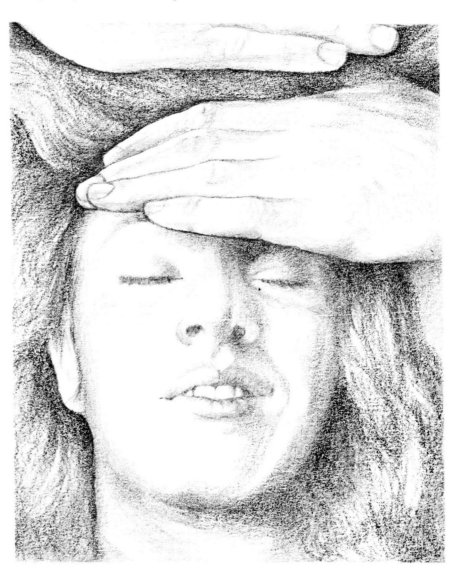

SPACING OUT

Place the hands on either side of the head, palms resting on the temples, fingertips resting on the 'third eye' area. Leave the hands here for one or two minutes in a light yet enclosing touch. To the person being 'spaced', it is as if all sudden movement and all sense of time is blocked off.

Tension often shows itself with a nagging headache or twitching nerves. A simple forehead press to close the third eye and eliminate tension can bring dramatic relief. Press down with a right hand, palm upon the centre of the forehead; use the left hand over the right to add extra pressure and to distribute the pressure evenly across the forehead; start by pushing down lightly, but let your strength become deeper and deeper. (If you are afraid of hurting the skull, ask your partner to tell you if it becomes too much). Reach maximum pressure slowly and allow it to last for about ten seconds. Then release just as gradually, allowing the palm, where it is in contact with the 'third eye' to be the last part of your hand to remain in touch. Then lift. This can be repeated several times.

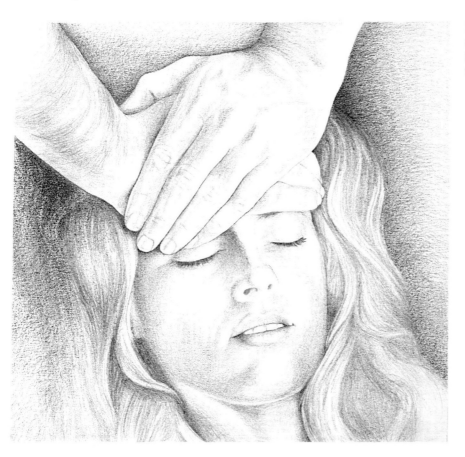

Third eye *Press down with the right hand, palm on the centre of the forehead. Add extra pressure with the left hand.*

One reason I enjoy going to the hairdresser's is the sensual experience of having my hair manipulated by the fingertips of the shampoo assistant. But it isn't necessary to anoint a head with slippery lather in order to give it a good time.

The frivolous follicles – a hair massage

Hair massage *Take small locks of hair between your thumb and forefingers and pull each clump GENTLY.*

Scalp manipulation *Support the head against your body then rotate the skin on the surface of the head with the flat of one hand.*

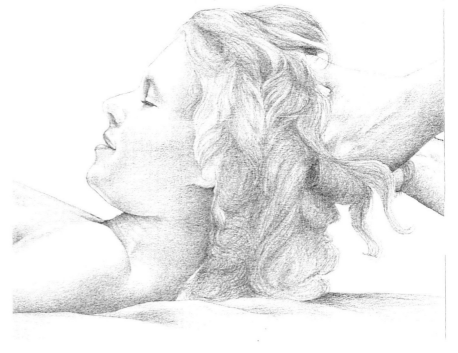

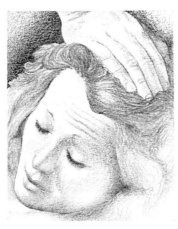

The Red Indians knew a thing or two when they removed their enemies' scalps. It wasn't just that their victims experienced a certain amount of pain (no, they didn't always die), but scalping also removed all the nerve endings. The victims therefore lost much of the sensation from the top of the head and suffered severe disorientation. Scalp manipulation aims at putting sensation *into* the head and incidentally can promote hair growth (reluctant baldies please note).

SCALP MANIPULATION

Cup the top of your partner's head with your full hand, supporting it against your body or with your other hand at the back of the skull. Press down with the massaging hand and rotate the skin stretched across the surface of the head. This may move very easily or it may seem tightly stretched. Tense people tend to posses tense scalps.

SCALP FRICTION

Once the whole head has been rotated this way, alter the stroke. Instead of rotating the skin itself, rotate the *hand* on the head, taking care not to pull the hair.

TUG OF LOVE

Take small locks of hair between your thumb and forefingers (using both hands at the same time) and pull each clump gently. This triggers off small but sensual prickings of feeling.

Using all the fingers, gently rake through the hair, across the surface of the scalp, as if your fingernails are a fine comb. Pull and swivel and swirl and rotate. Cover the entire head, not forgetting the sensitive nape of the neck. A fine-toothed nylon brush can provoke further scalp-tingling sensations.

THE FINGER COMB

Ask your partner to sit on a chair with his or her feet bare. Wrap each foot in a warm towel. You, kneeling in front of them, are equipped with two more towels, a large bowl of warm water and a bottle of liquid soap (peppermint flavour is very effective). Your partner's eyes should be closed throughout the exercise and on no account should your partner help in any way by moving his or her limbs; all such movement is *your* responsibility. The experience, for the person being pampered, is of helplessness, luxury and trust fulfilled, very like a baby's feelings.

The pampered foot – a foot massage

With one hand gently lift your partner's foot, while pulling the bowl of water into a central position in front of you with the other. Slowly slide the towel off their foot and gently immerse the foot into the water. Leave it there for two or three minutes, giving it time to thoroughly warm up.

Lift the foot from the water and move the bowl sideways to create a space in front of you. Then, move yourself forward into that space (still kneeling). Cover your knees with one of the extra towels, place your partner's foot on to the towel and immediately cover it in order to keep it warm for as long as possible.

Work enough soap into your hands to make them slippery, even lathery, then burrow into the towel, find the foot and sensitively apply the soap, coating the whole surface of the foot thoroughly. Using the thumbs of both hands, work small circling strokes over the foot, taking care not to massage hard on any bones because that hurts. Massage with the thumbs on the instep and pull gently down with the middle fingers on each side of the ankle in the space on either side of the Achilles tendon.

Tilting the foot on to the heel so that the sole is facing you, massage, with the thumbs, into the horny areas underneath. You may find you hold the foot by the heel with one hand and do the massage with the other. Naturally, large hands and small feet, or vice versa, will mean certain adaptations of technique.

Lovingly soap between each toe with a forefinger, rubbing (extra slowly) in and out of these very sensual areas. Using the thumb, pull it hard along the underside of the foot immediately below the toes, progressing from one side of the foot to the other. Don't be afraid of repeating strokes which seem specially successful.

Carry on caressing and kneading the entire foot, circling gently with the forefingers around the ankle bones.

Tug gently on each toe, grasping each toe between thumb and forefinger. Tug on the foot as a whole. Holding the foot with your left

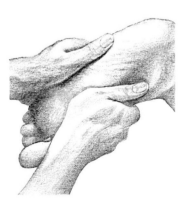

Foot massage *Tilting the foot, massage with your thumbs into the horny areas on the sole.*

hand at the back of the heel and the right hand across, pull slowly and firmly for a couple of seconds and then relax. Repeat two more times.

When the first foot has received at least ten minutes worth of attention, lift it carefully, pull the bowl back towards you, lower the foot into it, wash off the soap in the warm water and dry on a second warm towel.

Repeat the preceedings with the second foot.

Rag doll touch game

In this sequence of movements, your partner is treated as if they were a rag doll. It is unnecessary to remove any clothes for the exercise although your partner would feel comfortable with a bare neck.

While you visualise your partner as a doll who is new and unfamiliar, you also see yourself as a child exploring the doll for the first time. This exploration takes the shape of moving the doll's limbs at random to see what they do, what kind of shapes they make and how far they will stretch.

Your partner lies on his or her back and at no stage in the proceedings does he or she move. All movement is carried out by you. Spend about five minutes on each limb, moving it slowly and giving yourself time to find out how each one seems to function. Don't be afraid of gently *stretching* your partner's limbs.

Perhaps beginning with an arm, *manipulate* the finger, wrist, elbow and shoulder joints. Repeat with the other arm. Don't be afraid of *lifting* the limb to see what happens, but make sure you don't drop it.

Carry out similar movements on the legs. When lifting the knee it needs to be supported from underneath to avoid a sudden hurtful jerk when the leg is laid straight again. You can also try and 'walk' your partner by lifting and moving both legs, one after the other.

The head can be turned and tilted.

The arm could be treated to an *arm swing*. Sitting at your partner's side, pick up the arm nearest to you, holding it at the hand and the elbow. Hold it straight up with one hand and 'throw' it towards your other hand which should be hovering nearby ready to catch it (before it folds up and hits the floor with a thump). You establish a swing by throwing it backwards and forwards from one hand to the other. Each arm movement makes an arc and as you establish a rhythm the arc increases until it covers about a 90 degree angle. When you finish, catch the arm finally and lower it gently to the ground. Repeat with the other arm.

The chest lift – as a finishing off movement this is spectacular. Kneeling behind your partner's head, lean over and place your hands at your partner's waist, hooking them down the sides of their body and underneath. Pull your hands towards you, actually lifting them off the floor. As they progress towards you, your partner's body should arch towards you. When you reach the armpits, slowly slide your hands out and end the exercise.

Chest Lift

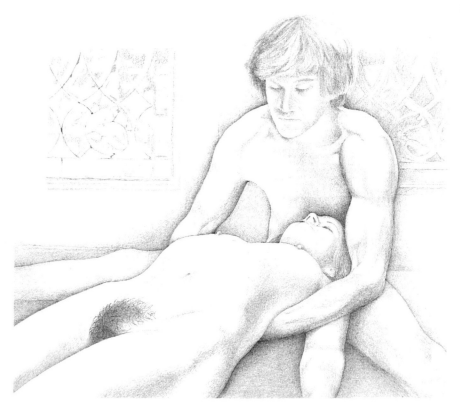

Non-threatening massages allow people to become intimate and to feel comfortable – a mirror to what happens in a healthy friendship. The only difference in a real friendship is that you would *each* take turns to give the other 'good strokes'. The next chapter takes us a little further along the route to intimacy.

Touch games people play

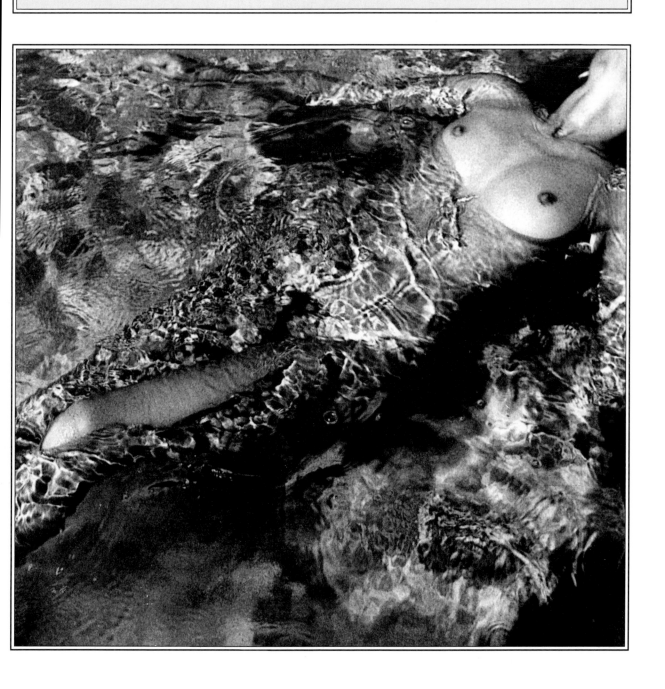

Nudity

It's a quantum leap from clothes to nudity, but if you want your partner to enjoy a massage fully they need to take their clothes off. And in order for them to feel comfortable in doing so *you* need to feel comfortable with nudity first.

I learned this lesson through a remarkable initial meeting with Ray Stubbs – a meeting startling for its lack of garments! I was visiting the institution where he teaches and, with a colleague, was walking towards the hall chatting. As we reached the relaxation area, a door to my left opened and out poured a stream of smiling, bouncy, naked people. At their head, wearing a large moustache and nothing else, carrying a bowl of soapy water, was a very thin man.

'Anne,' said the colleague, 'meet Ray'. Ray, smiling broadly, shifted the bowl to his left arm and formally shook hands with me. 'Nice to meet you.' He chatted and made small talk for five minutes, totally unconcerned about the fact that he didn't have a stitch on. Furthermore his students who, a week before had never done a massage in their lives, chatted and laughed beside us, glowing in the nude. They were covered in sweet-smelling massage oil and took it in turns to shower, shampoo and enjoy a hot bath. Much of their dressing activity was done right next to us. Such was their sense of comfort and acceptance of their nudity that I rapidly shared it. I didn't once feel embarrassed or inhibited myself – just initially amazed. I ended up wishing I could have shared what must have been a marvellous lesson.

On another occasion I and my partner were given a weekend holiday at a naturist village in the South of France. Our host, a man who in London was always impeccably dressed in a business suit, called for us on the first morning, stark naked. Since he was a large gentleman he seemed much *more* naked than I expected and somehow his presence made it even harder to take my own clothes off.

He proposed to show us around. Since it had been made clear that nudity wasn't compulsory, I acommpanied him to the beach wearing more clothes than usual. I was not comfortable. The more he showed us the shops, boutiques, even supermarkets where everyone strolled totally naked, the more overdressed I felt. As we reached the beach, I slowly but surely shed the layers until I ended up with a pair of sunglasses and a straw hat. Amongst the regular sunbathers who used this beach, we were told, was a priest and the nuns from a nearby convent – *all* naked. It was a revelation!

I learned a lot from these two experiences – not least of which was that the more comfortable those around you are with their naked body, the easier it gets for a newcomer to accept their own nudity.

This was particularly relevant when I began to take massage classes myself. In the first sessions, anticipating (I now realise) not the students' nervousness but my own, I hummed and haaed over what people might take off or leave on, with the result that I directed some complicated massage instruction through layers of clothes! That session didn't work out too well. We discovered rapidly the impossibility of giving a good back massage through someone's underwear.

As a result, I became matter-of-fact and directive. I began to pair people up so that they couldn't feel rejected if they were not chosen by their neighbour. I said loudly and clearly that while no one was forced to take off anything they didn't want to, a massage simply wouldn't work well through clothes.

These days, the most anyone leaves on is a pair of briefs and in the past eight years, only one person has ever opted out of the massage altogether. The difference is not in the type of person attending the class, but in the way *I* have learned to approach nudity.

What I particularly learned from Ray was how to make nudity normal for a massage. The technique is to believe it yourself. Nudity is easily accepted by clients, partners or friends when you believe it too. This doesn't have to be stated to them. In fact, it's better left unspoken. As long as you truly believe nudity is normal in massage, the weight of your beliefs will allow any instruction you give to be acceptable.

The best way to achieve this belief is to experience massage yourself, before you experiment on others. Seek out a friend who practises the skill as a sideline, or someone who already teaches massage, or even a professional masseur/se whom you pay for an all-over-body massage. You will be able to learn from these experiences not only what the massage feels like and how you handle nudity there, but also from the way in which masseur/se handles the situation.

The experience of massage

I was very lucky with my own first experience of massage. Back in the psychedelic '70s, I discovered that an enlightened acquaintance had started holding massage evenings for friends. Never famed for my diffidence I invited myself along. I was surprised to find the session included only me, but Jack seemed comfortable with this so I relaxed too. The massage was sensitively done – so good in fact that it made a profound impression; I have never forgotten it.

So much in this first experience surprised me. For example, having my hands stroked and manipulated was one of the friendliest sensations I'd ever known. What grew out of this (and the rest of the massage) was warmth, gratitude, even affection for the man who had given me such a wonderful time even though he was only an acquaintance. I hadn't understood before how anyone might acquire such intimate feelings for someone they hardly knew.

Three years later I experienced the same affection for Ray in our first massage session. I learned from these moments of fortune a great deal about myself and about others. My immediate thoughts were, if I could feel so strongly towards someone I didn't really know, how much more would I feel towards a lover? Subsequent experiments demonstrated that my strong feelings amplified dramatically when I carried out a similar massage session *with* a lover.

I understood that concentrated sessions of touch are an adult equivalent to the childhood sensations of being mothered, nurtured, comforted, cared for and valued. All these impressions fed into my brain while the touching fed into my body. And those superb massages managed to let me feel like a lucky child again, handled and loved in the same way as when I was a baby.

Such richness of caress awakened me to the realisation of how starved I was of touch in the normal pattern of life. I don't think this experience is uncommon. Once we reach adolescence most of us crave for loving touch even if we don't know just what it is that troubles our puzzled bodies.

Sociologists Skipper and McCaghy studied thirty-five strippers and found that some 60 per cent of them came from broken or unstable homes in which the father was in some way inadequate. Their conclusions were that the strippers, in baring their bodies, might be asking for the love and affection they hadn't received from their fathers. In other words they were (theoretically?) making their skin available for touch contact *which they needed*. What seems equally likely to me is that these women also missed the caresses they would have or should have received from their *mothers*!

Ray Stubbs, an astute American, has recognised that his fellows suffer particularly from skin starvation. As a result he and his partner, Walter Wilding, set up a skin-to-skin service of a sort unheard of in this country. Called The Secret Garden Ceremony, he and Walter created an extraordinary routine which reads like a touch-starved person's dream.

The Secret Garden Ceremony

Ray's formula is one which could be happily copied by couples. One entire session could be devoted to the woman; another separate time could be reserved for the man. The Secret Garden Ceremony inspires trust, pleasure and feelings of sheer luxury. It is not a massage, although massage is included. It is (in many ways literally) a feast. It could be used as a lead-in to more serious massage sessions, or, if it seems ultra-daring, it could become an intense follow-up to a straightforward massage.

Since the emphasis is on sensuality, it is important to arrange the atmosphere of The Secret Garden to blend in with the sensuality of the exercise. Ideally it should be carried out on velvet mattresses in an orchid-filled hothouse with non-stop Albinoni playing in the background before you jump into your own personal, exclusive hot bath. Since few of us have access to private botanical gardens, we may have to do with indoor plants in the living room, easy access to the bathroom and exclusive use of the home for the duration of the session.

This is what Ray and Walter do. The client, once she has booked Ray and Walter's time, arranges to meet them at her own apartment or, if there are likely to be inconveniences, at a motel room with bathroom for the afternoon. Ray and Walter, on arrival, ensure that the room is warm, the telephone off the hook and that, amongst their apparatus, is included a feast of tropical fruits.

1. The first part of The Secret Garden Ceremony consists of these two handsome young men softly bathing their client (usually but not always a woman), rubbing her with bath oil, soaping her gently, even getting into the bath with her and cradling her lovingly in the water. Please note, at no time is there *any* sex included. In fact Ray makes a point of stating this at the onset, so that his clients' expectations of the experience are realistic.

2. Once she is rosy and relaxed, the young men, both naked themselves (part of the visual feast) feed their by now laid-back bather with peeled sweet grapes, titbits of fresh pineapple, spoonfuls of ripe mango, huge Californian strawberries (prepared in advance). No matter if the juices roll down her – it is a simple matter of rubbing the dribbles down her skin and into the perfumed water of the bath.

Once she has soaked and relaxed enough, she is helped out of the bath and lovingly wrapped in a fluffy, warm towel. Then the three move to the main room where the client is lingeringly dried as if she were an infant. At no time does she have to move a finger.

3. The next stage is to pamper her skin. The client lies down on a firm mattress covered with more of the warm fluffy towels and, rather like the Queen of Sheba, is stroked with peacock feathers. If this weren't enough she is next rubbed all over with velvet and finally with a soft fur mitt.

4. The teasing and rubbing is merely a 'vorspeiser', an appetite stimulator, which hints of wonders to come. Sometimes, at this stage, Ray plays quiet tunes on his flute and then, using the music as a means of linking ideas, talks his client through a series of guided fantasies. Afterwards Walter encourages the client to describe what she saw during Ray's descriptions.

5. Now for the massage. This is what it has all been leading up to. First there has been the feast of skin nurtured by water. Then there was the feast of eyes, with the view of the two beautiful young men and the gorgeous looking tropical fruit, then there are further skin sensations in the warm towels and beneath the peacock feathers. The exotic fruit proves the feast of the tastebuds and next there is the internal feast of the ears and mind with the fantasy story.

Now comes the banquet. A surfeit of hands slips around her body. Ray and Walter caress and massage every part of their client. They smooth and glide, stroke and swoop, creating waves of sensation.

6. Finally, when the happy client is tingling in every pore, the massage is rounded off with the energy sweep. (For details about

whole-body massage see pages 29–35 and 42–50, for details of the energy sweep, see page 59.) Every ounce of excess sensitivity is swept away out of the limbs and head, and the client is filled with a feeling of well-being. It is not sexual. She does not have an erotic climax (unless one happens spontaneously), nor is she intended to have one. What she does enjoy is an ultimate awareness of her bodily reflexes in a childlike way and the impression of being completely cared for.

It is no accident that Ray and Walter begin their skin-to-skin service with a warm bath. Many lovers discover by happy chance how immersion in warm water enhances skin responsiveness. In water the skin acquires extra properties, becoming smooth, slippery and sinuous.

Hot water therapy

Floating in the bath undoubtedly brings back subconscious memories of floating deep inside the shelter of mother's womb – the only totally safe experience we will know in our lifetime. Harking back to it, may help restore some of our inner peace.

Californians among others are readily aware, of the anti-stress value of hot-water relaxation. The Institute for the Advanced Study of Human Sexuality in San Francisco is a bona fide centre for further education within the United States' education system, licensed to grant degrees for appropriate academic work. Inside the Institute, just off the main foyer, is a huge redwood tub, big enough to seat several people comfortably. This is a giant jacuzzi and is kept on a continual hot bubble.

It is available to everyone working within the Institute. So strongly do the directors of the organisation feel about the value of touch that staff and students are encouraged to relax. The hot tub is part of this encouragement. At 4 pm most afternoons, the presidents of the college, the Reverend Ted McIlvenna and the dean, Dr Wardell Pomeroy, can be viewed taking their teabreak there.

Indeed, the Reverend Ted feels so strongly about the therapeutic effect of water on skin that he actually teaches sex therapy to young couples *in* the pool. He gets some pleasing (and pleased) results. Couples, in the relaxing yet stimulating water environment, regress to their childhood, remembering what it was like to play in the bath as kids. They have fun, they splash each other, they kiss and cuddle and suddenly sex therapy becomes an easier game.

Touch games

Games are specifically used in California as therapy. They are used to get communication established, to teach people how to talk, to unblock frustrations, to repair marital damage, to bring back some 'sparkle' into a dulled sex-life or even to get sex going in the first place. Many of these games have their roots in infancy and are used by therapists such as Irene Kassorlas, William Hartman and Marilyn Fithian. The following are some of their best known strategies.

The foot bath

This is the same as the Pampered Foot described in the previous chapter. Couples take it in turns to bath and caress each other's feet.

The hair sweep

Here couples sensitively wash, comb and brush each other's hair, paying great emphasis on being slow and patient.

Spoons

In this exercise the couple lies together 'back to front', fitting together like a pair of spoons. The one at the back has to synchronise breathing to match the one at the front. It can be deeply relaxing, almost hypnotic, when getting in rhythm with each other in this way.

Mirror on the wall

Standing nude in front of a full-length mirror, you touch every part of yourself from the top of your head down to the bottom of your feet, including the genitals. At the same time you say out loud what you like and dislike about the parts of your body and how they feel when you touch them.

The next section of this exercise is to repeat it on the following day in front of a partner. Don't speak at all during the touching and looking, but share your feelings afterwards. The partner should do the same.

The final section of 'mirror on the wall' is for you *both* to repeat the exercise on a third day. Only this time, say what immediately comes into your head about each part of your body and how it feels. How we regard our bodies affects our sensuality. Sharing our fears and inhibitions with a partner can do much to help us accept how we look and ultimately how we experience touch.

Hand play

Stroke, clasp, rub and caress each other's hands for ten minutes.

Cuddling

Spend fifteen minutes cuddling each other.

Finger tipping

Spend fifteen minutes running your fingertips over your partner's back while they do the same for you.

Good sensuality is built on unhurried times together when we establish trust through touch. These games return us to our early steps of learning-to-trust. Deliberate eroticism and genital touch are excluded to give us the chance to relax and enjoy.

The games don't have to be used as therapy. They can be used as methods of getting to know someone. Some people may prefer to discard the more sexual exercises in order to concentrate on something simple.

Those already in an intimate relationship, however, may feel the need for something more. Hartman and Fithian's game, Plus Three–Minus Three may provide it.

Plus Three–Minus Three

One partner sits nude in a comfortable armchair while the other stands then later kneels in front of them. The chairless partner strokes the seated one on specific areas of their skin, not more than two inches in diameter, with one finger, once or twice. These strokes begin at the top of the head, work their way down the body to the soles of the feet. After every stroke, the stroking partner stops and the seated one rates how those strokes feel. They are rated on a Plus Three–Minus Three scale.

If, for example, strokes on the forehead feel acceptable but not special, they might be rated as nought. If strokes along the side of the breast seemed very sensual, you might rate these as plus three. If a touch was uncomfortable or even unpleasant, it would take you into the minuses. And if a particular stroke felt sensational, it might go way over the top to plus ten!

Although the exercise sounds contrived when described, it is not when carried out. You need to *feel* it to understand its worth.

David and Caroline were in therapy for a sex life which had diminished to a point of non-existence. They found, on playing Plus Three–Minus Three, that Caroline experienced sensual feeling for the first time since she was a child. David, on the other hand, felt, for the first time in the marriage, that he was both an attractive and a responsive person. The most important understanding to come out of these sessions was Caroline's observation, 'I've been enabled to find something sexual in David I've never found in any other man. I was physically moved. It's what I would call real eroticism.' Their relationship *didn't* suddenly blast off into a rocket-like explosiveness, but doing the exercises gave them a positive starting point for further therapy.

Although the game includes touching the genitals it is not designed for sexual arousal. The main aims of Plus Three–Minus Three are to teach people about their own and their partner's body, to communicate about what does and doesn't feel good and to have fun.

Plus Three–Minus Three takes us a long way past the initial nervousness of beginning a massage for the first time, but some people are also helped come to terms with nudity by playing the game. It is quite possible too to enjoy the exercise when it is carried out with a friend instead of a lover.

Pleasant surroundings, warmth and sweet smells help make a massage enjoyable. At the very least warmth is a must. If the room is cold, prepare it beforehand and, if necessary, keep the heater on for the duration of the massage.

Do *not* massage on a bed – it is too bouncy. Use a massage table or the floor with a towel or blanket spread over it.

Warm the massage oil beforehand. One way of doing this is to float the bottle of oil in a warm bath, so that both you and the bottle reach the right temperature.

Ensure that your hands are both clean and warm before beginning. Cold hands will tense up your partner and any tiny piece of grit that may be on your hands will be felt like a piercing scratch during the session.

Remove any jewellery which may affect your partner; this includes rings, watches, even necklaces which may trail across their body.

Since you need to move easily, it is sensible to wear few but stretchy garments.

Keep your nails trimmed so that they cannot scratch your partner.

When you start applying the oil make sure you rub it into *your own hands* first before passing it on to your partner's skin. Do *not* empty the massage oil directly on to them because this provides an unpleasant shock. When initially applying the oil, do so in short, rapid strokes. Any time the oil wears off and your partner's skin seems dry, apply more oil. When you do the massage proper, always SLOW IT DOWN.

Once the massage proper begins do not lose touch with your partner's body again until the end of the massage. This means, that even if you re-apply oil you do so while still keeping the back of one hand resting on their body.

If you are worried about oil spilling on the carpet, make sure it is placed on a towel where it is unlikely to be knocked over. Some people like to pour their oil into a saucer, feeling it is less accident-prone. Don't forget – keep the massage SLOW.

Preparing for a massage

All the exercises mentioned so far are a preparation for that culmination of deliberate touch – a body massage. In the last section of this chapter, therefore, eleven basic strokes to be used in a back massage are described.

Back massage

The back is the best part of the anatomy to begin on when doing body massage for the first time. It is less sexually threatening than the front, where breasts and genitals may present obstacles. The buttocks may be mildly threatening but the way to deal with your inhibitions is to remind yourself firmly that if they are left out they *feel* left out and the massage becomes inadequate. If you want to reinforce this attitude, the best way to do so is to have a back massage yourself where the buttocks are deliberately left out. You won't like it.

1. Circling

Place the palms of both hands on the shoulders and move them in circles, firmly outwards and away from the backbone, progressing down the back, along the sides of the body, until you reach the buttocks.

Continue circling on down the buttocks until you reach the upper part of the legs where you reverse the process and go back up the body.

When you return to the shoulders, encompass the top part of the arms, and end by returning across the shoulders to the neck where your thumbs should naturally penetrate the hairline, and perform a little individual massage of their own.

The circling stroke can be carried out over the back six times, and, of course, the pressure of the stroke can be varied. As you grow more experienced, your fingers will sense the depth that your friend will enjoy. On the last circling session, finish below the buttocks.

2. The glide

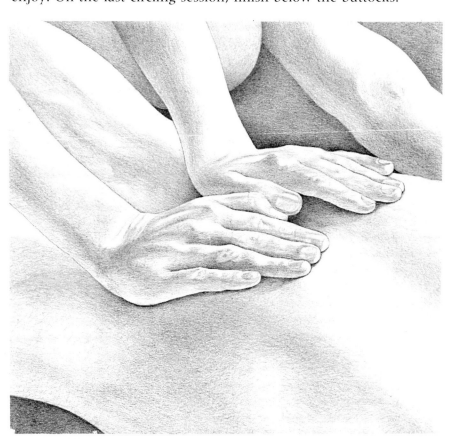

Glide *The weight of your body drives your hands, palms flat on either side of the spine, from the buttocks, right up to the shoulders.*

The most spectacular part of any massage. Place your hands on the lowest part of your friend's bottom with the palms flat and the fingers pointing towards the head. Then, with the weight of your body directed from the solar plexus, start pushing both hands up along the spine, taking as long as you like.

This is a heavy stroke as you are actually leaning on your partner. And your partner experiences this as a sense of overwhelming ripple, like a wave that flows directly along the back and threatens to engulf the head.

When you reach the shoulders and neck, lightly bring your hands down again to the buttocks and recommence.

It is important not to break contact with your partner. If you have to apply extra oil, try to keep part of your body in touch.

3. Swimming

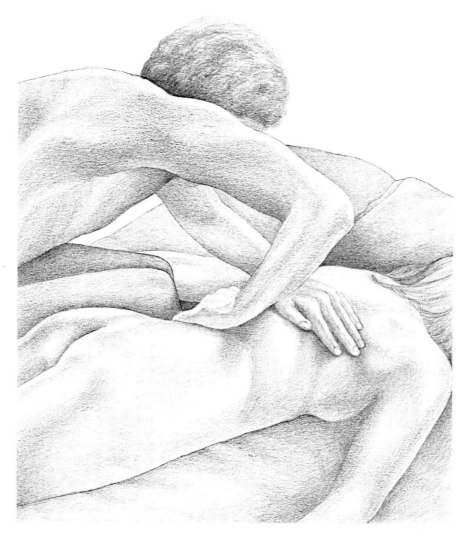

Swimming *Move your hands in circles, close together but in opposite directions to each other.*

Swimming

The hands, using the palms, move in circles close together but in opposite directions to each other, taking on a kind of swimming sensation. This can be carried out up and down all the fleshy parts of the body, including the buttocks.

It is a good idea to include the buttocks as often as possible, as this can be one of the most sensual zones of the back. Touching the bottom can bring on prickles of delicious sensation to the breast, the head and the genitals.

4. Weighting

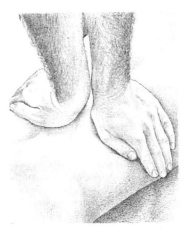

This is aimed to eliminate the tension that many people experience in the lower back. Sitting by your partner's side, place both hands on either side of the spine, just below the waistline, with fingers pointing sideways and down towards the hips. Lean heavily on your hands, applying the pressure evenly and allowing the force of your body alone to move your hands apart and down, as slowly as possible. They will slide slowly apart. Move your hands down the back slightly and repeat the same movement from the waist down to the area just above the tail of the spine (coccyx) as many times as your partner wants. The effect is of moving the strain out from the spinal column and away through the sides of the body.

Weighting *Place both hands on either side of the spine, just below the waist, fingers pointing sideways. Lean heavily on them, allowing your body weight to move the hands apart and down the sides of your partners body.*

5. Thumb over thumb

Working with both thumbs on the lower back, make short, rapid, alternate strokes with each thumb, moving up the buttocks towards the waist. Carry this on up the right-hand side of the body to the shoulders, repeat on the left-hand side, and finish off by concentrating again on the buttocks.

6. Cobblestones

Sitting by your partner's side, place your right hand on the base of the spine, fingers pointing towards the head, with the left hand over it. Then slowly glide over the spine itself. This has a curious bumpy motion like driving over cobblestones.

Come back down again at the same speed. As you come down, dig two fingers into the indentations on either side of the spine, raising your right hand slightly so that the maximum pressure can be applied. Do these strokes three times.

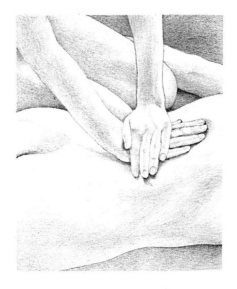
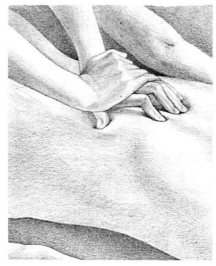

Cobblestones *Place your right hand on the base of the spine, fingers pointing towards the head, with the left hand over the right. Then glide the hands up the spine.*

As you return down the spine dig two fingers into the indentations on either side of the spine, raising your right hand slightly so that the maximum pressure can be applied.

By hooking the thumb into the space beneath the shoulder-blade you can create a curious feeling of helplessness. This may be difficult to do if your partner is muscular and the best way to seek out the hollow beneath the shoulder-blade is to lift his or her arm up and fold it across their back. This brings the shoulder-blade into sharp relief. Hook your thumb into the hollow beneath the shoulder-blade and pull it through and up towards the neck slowly. Do this three or four times, and then gently place the arm back on the ground, and do the same with the other arm and shoulder-blade.

8. With both hands flat, fingers pointing towards the head, start at the top of the shoulders pulling your thumbs, at a deep pressure, down the hollows on either side of the spine, till you reach the buttocks. You can repeat this exercise three times, on each occasion varying the pressure of the stroke.

9. When you reach the buttocks on the third repeat, make a variation of the glide by putting your full weight behind your thumbs and glide heavily up your partner's back, finishing in the hairline.

Using rapid pulling strokes on one arm at a time with the flat of both hands, cover the area from shoulder to wrist. Pulling strokes are hand over hand flat strokes that pull the skin in one direction, in the case of the limbs starting near the trunk and descending to either hands or feet.

Hand to hand deep palming in circles. This consists of placing the flat of *your* hand on the flat of your *partner's* hand and kneading around the centre of their hand with the bony areas of yours.

7. Thumb pressure strokes

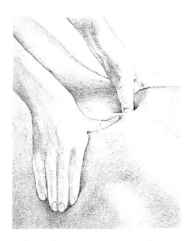

Thumb pressure strokes *Glide your thumbs up your partners back, on each side of the spine, putting your full weight behind them.*

10. The arms and hands

Hand over hand *Rapid pulling strokes, one at a time with the whole hand cover the area from shoulder to wrist.*

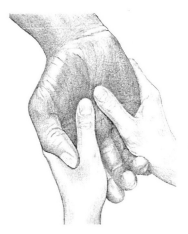

Deep palming *With both your thumbs, knead the fleshy parts of your partners hands.*

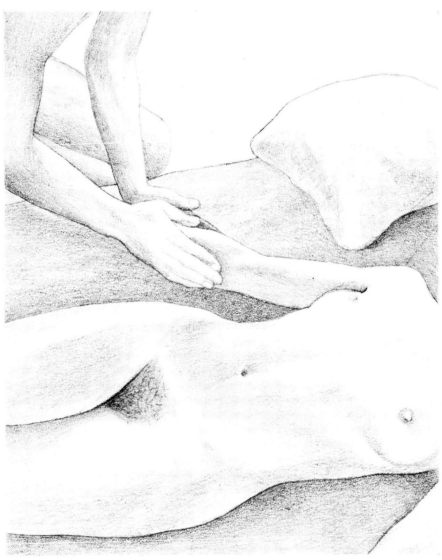

With both your thumbs, knead the fleshy parts of your partner's hands. This can be difficult if he or she is thin.

Very lightly and slowly, pull your forefinger down between each of your partner's fingers towards the palm, till all four finger spaces have been caressed.

Using the finger nails, rake the palm and the wrist.

All these movements should be repeated on the other arm and hand.

11. Finishing off

With both hands, grasp your partner at the top of the arms and very slowly pull your hands down the arms, slowing down even more at the hands and at the fingertips. Delay breaking finger contact till the last possible second and even then keep one finger touching for longer than the others before finally letting go. Keeping that finger contact somehow retains the energy and warmth generated between you. It's a poignant moment.

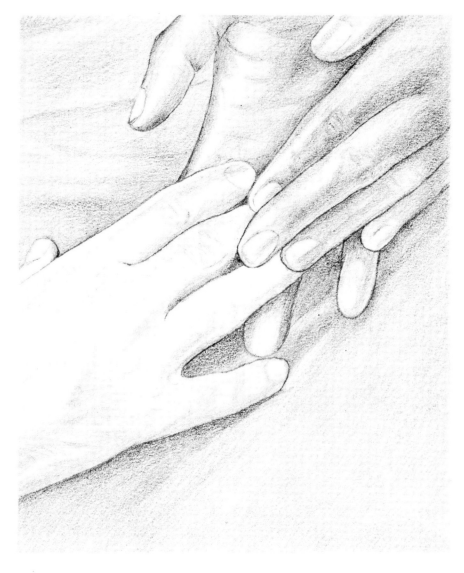

Finishing off *Delay breaking finger contact for the last possible second and even then, keep one finger touching for longer than the others.*

These eleven strokes are the basis of a back massage. Their sensual effect depends on the type of pressures used, the use of the finger nails on the erogenous zones and the subtlety of where you place your caresses.

The pleasure of touch

Familiarity with touch can actually change our lifestyle. Many of us have experienced that moment with a dear friend when we like them so much we ache to give them a hug, but somehow we don't – we are too inhibited. When we hold back, we feel empty and inadequate as a result. We don't possess the courage to express our inner selves.

Getting comfortable with touch enables us to break through the inhibitions and it doesn't take a degree in mathematics to deduce that a friendship is enriched by showing your warm feelings. When my girlfriend, Mary, broke up with her man I was pleased to be able to hold her tight when she needed, in grief, to be held. Before my 'touch conscience' was awakened, I doubt if I would have been able to do that.

There are a number of ways which we can learn to be more demonstrative and get ourselves used to the idea of touch in everyday life. The following are just a few:

1. When you say hello to someone, shake their hand.
2. When you say goodbye, touch their arm.
3. If you are talking with a friend, make a point of touching them on the arm when emphasizing something in the conversation.
4. Discuss this book with a friend.
5. When walking with a friend, put your arm through theirs for a while. Alternatively, and if appropriate, put an arm around their waist for a short time.
6. If you feel warm towards someone give them a farewell hug.
7. Start kissing your friends hello and goodbye.

These are small gestures but your friends will warm towards you. It is very pleasant to feel liked and that is what you demonstrate by this type of behaviour.

Touch and survival

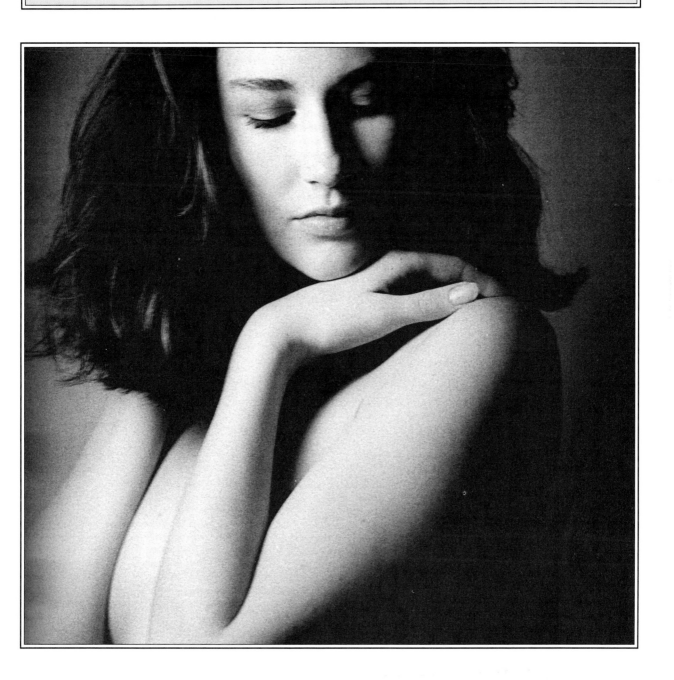

Childhood touch

Survival, I have suggested, can be a matter of 'touch and go'. On page 8 touch was shown to be vital for the survival of babies in orphanages and there has been some fascinating neurological studies to discover the reasons why. While I would hate to liken the human race in any way to laboratory rats, the fact remains that some of the research done on rats may well have relevance to the species of man. In the early 1950s rats were the subject of a survey done by Dr John D. Benjamin of the University of Colorado, Denver, USA. The survey studied the effects caresses and cuddles had on twenty rats (compared with twenty other rats who did *not* receive such tactile stimulation.)

'It sounds silly,' one investigator is reported to have remarked, 'but the petted rats learned faster and grew faster.' Some findings from this experiment were that the handled rats tended to be more exploratory, more confident, less intimidated by the testers, grew a heavier brain with greater development in certain parts of it, showed greater liveliness and curiosity, became more advanced in body growth, were less prone to illness, recovered from physical shock much more quickly, learned more quickly, became sexually more responsive and more sexually developed than the rats in the control study. All this from strokes and cuddles.

If the work with rats may be related to human, we can assume that the more physically stroked and caressed we are as infants, the more neurological development we are likely to generate within our bodies and the more tactile our behaviour will eventually become.

Indeed, research along the same line of thinking but with children deprived of maternal touch in institutions, showed them to be mentally disadvantaged, to have about half the bone growth of a normal child and invariably to possess skin of a deep pallor instead of a healthy pink colour.

One of the spin-offs of receiving tactile pleasure is that we get to feel we deserve it. Physical caress enables us to feel good about ourselves; it allows us to think we are valuable as people. We also like the individuals who give us pleasing strokes. When you like someone you tend to make an effort to please them too. And so the effect of good touch can spiral. Good touch can make us better spouses, parents, friends and relations.

The power of touch

Good touch allows relationships to form *and* survive. It makes it more likely that we remain happily married, that there is affection between parent and child. It enables relationships to pick up if they've been going through a bad patch; it renews the feelings of caring between two people. This is as true of two young people doing a therapeutic massage as it is of an older married couple.

We began in the first chapter with fun and games and going back to childhood. Now we continue with working at a relationship, experimenting with different types of touching and taking the risk of going a little further with touch exercises.

Once past the first stages of a relationship it is common to meet with problems which at first we perhaps didn't perceive. Take people, for instance, who have never received much touch in the past. Some of these unfortunates actually recoil from touch. Their skin is 'tight', resembling a body armour. There are special types of touch helpful for these tense individuals, designed to unlock both the 'armour' and the feelings that have been trapped inside them.

Rolfing is a type of deep massage developed by Dr Ida Rolf of Colorado, USA. In this massage, a deep pressure is applied along the muscles, tendons and knotted tissue of the entire torso, legs, arms, head and neck. Be warned that rolfing can be extremely painful to begin with, but by freeing muscles which may always have been taut the individual can even feel painful childhood experiences loosen and subsequently can feel pleasurable sensation fo the first time.

A similar method has been successfully used on autistic children where they are given a 'maternal and soft' massage to begin with, then a very deep pressure massage which begins to hurt. The children may react to this with protest, but they are reassured this is the 'right' reaction to have. Then they are given more soothing and mothering touch as further reassurance. They learn from this the ability to distinguish between pleasure and pain, something they couldn't previously separate. Learning to separate such basic sensations is the beginning of their route to normality.

The Dolman School in Philadelphia, USA, teaches parents to use similar methods of massage, limb exercise and enforced crawling with brain damaged or autistic children in order to imprint in their brains the appropriate signals and responses. They are teaching the children normal tactile sensations which enable them to become more normal themselves. Similar methods have been used in the treatment of schizophrenic patients, including some fascinating stories of breakthroughs with catatonic schizophrenics who responded instantly to sympathetic touch after years of being locked inside their own heads.

Most of us however are not catatonic, schizophrenic or autistic. We may not even be aware that there are gaps in our childhood experience. But if, for minor reasons, we didn't enjoy pleasure and comfort through touch with a parent when we most yearned for it, then perhaps somewhere in the brain, small parts of our innermost self have been locked away and labelled 'unacceptable'. Liberating these baby mis-beliefs or perhaps experiencing a deep need gratified by touch for the first time can be a moving occasion. Touch teaches us to love and be loved.

Love is a strong word, but a good massage can provoke strong feeling. There are people who cherish little chunks of true affection for Ray Stubbs, for example, all over America, Canada and Europe — myself included. Massage is one of the fastest ways of becoming intimate with someone *if you want it to be so.*

Touch and depression

Massage gives some people hope where none existed before. Take Lily and Heather, for example, two deeply depressed women who participated in a couple of the women's sexuality workshops that I run.

Lily was a 20-year-old German student living in this country. She was depressed and suicidal. The day we did the massage in her group had been a specially bad day for her. She had telephoned earlier and said, among other things, that life wasn't worth living. Later that evening, during the massage, she discovered that first she could actually tolerate someone touching her, and secondly the touch felt so good, friendly and comforting she was hopeful once more. During the weeks which followed, she changed drastically. She bought new clothes, looked ten times healthier, the depression lifted and shortly afterwards she stopped seeing her psychiatrist. The massage had been a turning point. Two years later the depression hadn't returned and she was about to marry.

Heather was in a second group. She was a 36-year-old South African who had lived in this country since she was 20. She was almost too depressed to speak. She lived on her own, never left her bedsitter except to go to a robot-like job in the Post Office. In the space of a half an hour massage in the group she changed from a dumpy, rather plain girl into a glowing and appealing woman. The transformation continued throughout the course. Her depression didn't clear as rapidly as Lily's, but there was less and she coped with what remained much better.

She also described the group massage as finding hope. When I again heard from her she had changed her job; then, eighteen months later, she decided to emigrate to Canada to join her sister and start a new life there.

Both these women had got out of touch with themselves, partly through being deprived of physical touch (Lily hadn't dated anyone for two years, Heather for four). Because both were living away from their native countries, neither were able to seek comfort from their families. It is easy to believe, if no one ever touches you, that you are simply unworthy of love. In itself, that is too depressing to handle.

Self-love

A common denominator amongst the women who attend sexuality workshops is a profound lack of self-esteem. Perhaps like Lily and Heather they haven't been touched for years. Or like Deborah they don't feel important enough to be loved so they don't seek relationships with men (or women). Or they feel that because they do not instantly respond to their partner's touch they are a failure.

Outside the workshops in everyday life, there are men and women who feel so unloved that their prickly feelings about themselves get transmitted to others. Battered wives number amongst these. Many of them have a history of coming from a battered home themselves. Family touch to them is painful touch.

Men and women who pressurise their partners for sex continually may not actually be highly sexed; they may instead be saying, 'I don't feel very loveable. Show me that you love me.' Husbands who are jealous of their own children may resent the care and attention their offspring receive and grieve unknowingly for the loss of that same care and attention for themselves.

The answer to many of these problems is to learn to love yourself. You should have learnt this in childhood, but perhaps the right input was not available at the right time. It is harder to absorb new teaching in adulthood, but nevertheless possible. As shown with brain-damaged people, touch is one of the most direct methods of achieving this.

Self-touch

In Kate's case self-massage turned out to be an important factor of change. Kate's relationship with her man was unsatisfactory, she wasn't orgasmic, neither did she feel in control at work although her job was a senior one. A combination of self-massage and simple assertion skills enabled Kate to make massive changes. She became orgasmic, found a more sympathetic partner and dealt with issues at work with new confidence.

Kate was so impressed with the self-massage that she went on to study touch in depth. Her new massage skills add a very satisfactory postscript to her story. Working as a social worker, Kate regularly visited old people and decided to use her newly learned massage techniques to give them a treat. It seems incredible but using massage is a new departure for a social worker and in doing so Kate was breaking through a number of barriers, some of them taboos. The validation for her directness lay in the old peoples' response; they welcomed her visits with plaintive eagerness. Some of them hadn't been hugged or cuddled for years. While her colleagues still employed more verbal methods of care, Kate nurtured her clients with her hands.

Self-massage – a three-day routine

Day One

1. The first step is to start feeling comfortable with your own body. Take a bath, soap yourself slowly and sensually including the parts that might get forgotten, like between the toes, around and on the genitals, inside the navel.

2. Dry yourself with a warm bathtowel and move to a ready-warmed bedroom. Anoint yourself with sweet smelling massage oil and slowly rub this into the skin. Take your time, enjoy yourself, get to know your body. Notice the difference textures of skin and muscle. Learn to recognise which parts of the body feel good and which parts not so comfortable. But *don't* include the genitals.

Day Two
Carry out the previous two exercises, only this time you may include the genitals. Stroke and cream and caress them just as you do the rest of your body, noticing where good feeling comes from. Learn to build on these feelings. Give your body a treat.

Day Three
1. Begin as previously but concentrate more on the erogenous areas than before. If your nipples feel wonderful, then smooth and caress them. If your thighs tingle with good feeling, then help them tingle some more. If your genitals feel great, carry on nourishing that sensation.

2. Spend one hour doing exactly what you most want to do. This time is for your benefit and no one elses. If it means rolling on a sheepskin rug naked while listening to Wagner and reading *The Story of O* then enjoy, enjoy.

Self touch *Anoint yourself with sweet-smelling massage oil and slowly rub this in. Enjoy yourself, get to know your body.*

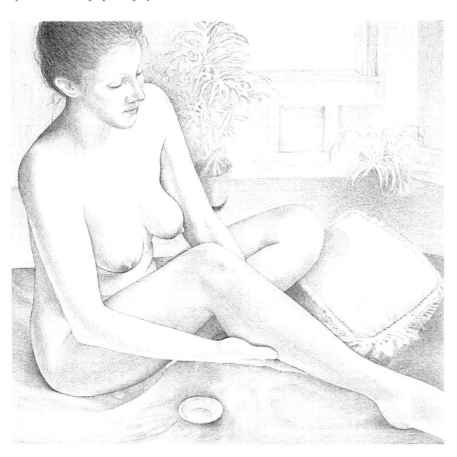

In the front line – a chest and abdomen massage

The following massage (on the chest and abdomen) is the next step in enlarging a touch repertoire that already includes touch games, self-touch and a back massage. It will be specially enjoyed by couples who have completely shed their inhibitions about nudity, couples in personal relationships who have established firm trust and caring between them and couples in a long-term relationship who are looking for emotional high-spots in their life to act as a method of continuation. The survival of a loving but possibly low-key affair may depend on bringing something extra into it. Enhanced sensuality is a delightful and effective aid.

Some couples in long-time relationships are aware of an unspoken, almost unconscious ache for something not received. Massage at the hands of someone you love can salve that ache.

If the buttocks seem a barrier to back massage, the breasts and genitals are undoubtedly the obstacles in a front massage. One couple in sex therapy remained transfixed by the back for six months, an indication of how each of them feared the other's sexuality. Some professional masseurs/ses won't touch the breasts on grounds of decency. Yet anyone who experiences a front massage which leaves the breasts out will tell you how incomplete such a routine feels.

One reason the breasts arouse such anxiety is because they seem vulnerable; partners are afraid of hurting them. Yet the secret of good breast massage lies in *how* you touch. And in order to know how, you need information about the breasts first. Is your partner pregnant? Has she recently had a baby? Is she breastfeeding? Is there some other physical reason for possessing specially sensitive breasts? These are some of the conditions where touch can be painful, if it is not done very gently and carefully. But most women like breast massage and regret the lack of it. So investigate before you start.

Women who have had breast surgery may have very mixed feelings about a chest and abdomen massage. For some it is immensely reassuring to know that someone is happy about looking at and even touching their scar tissue. For others this may be so traumatic that a chest massage is out of the question. Women who are able to take the risk often find this a very emotional and rewarding experience indeed, to feel their surgically altered chest being caressed and cared for.

The male chest isn't such a problem. Women may be interested to hear that some (but not all) male nipples are often specially sensitive and are sometimes so responsive that the entire body reacts. The male genitals, however, may be a 'no-go' area. Some men are afraid of getting an erection; some women are also afraid he will. It should reassure both sexes to understand that an erection doesn't 'get in the way' of a massage. It should be seen merely as an indicator of whole body arousal, *not* necessarily of sexual urgency.

Female genitals don't pose such a threat since most front massage is done kneeling at the side of the body or at the head which means the female genitalia don't give the impression of representing a prime target area.

Ideally a front massage follows on from a back massage. Help your partner to move on to his or her back since it can be quite a shock to

Where to begin

move when you've been lulled into a state of blissful relaxation. Help him or her to roll over slowly. If, for any reason, there is a wait between front and back massage, cover your partner with a towel or sheet since he or she will get chilled easily.

Some teachers begin by massaging the abdomen and then graduating upwards to the chest. But the abdomen is a sensitive area and if touched too hard or too softly it can react with irritation which naturally affects further reaction. The abdomen is less likely to be irritated by a session which begins at the shoulders, then goes across the chest before finally concentrating on the abdomen. The rest of the body will be prepared to expect a good sensation.

CHEST AND ABDOMEN STROKE

Kneel at your partner's head. Rub plenty of massage oil into your hands, then place them, palms down, on the middle of the chest, your fingers pointing towards the feet and the heel of your hands just below the collar bone. Your thumbs should be lightly touching each other.

Glide both hands slowly forward and down your partner's body, pressing firmly on the chest and less firmly across the abdomen. Keep your hands together until you reach the pubis or, if you cannot stretch that far, as far down the abdomen as you can manage.

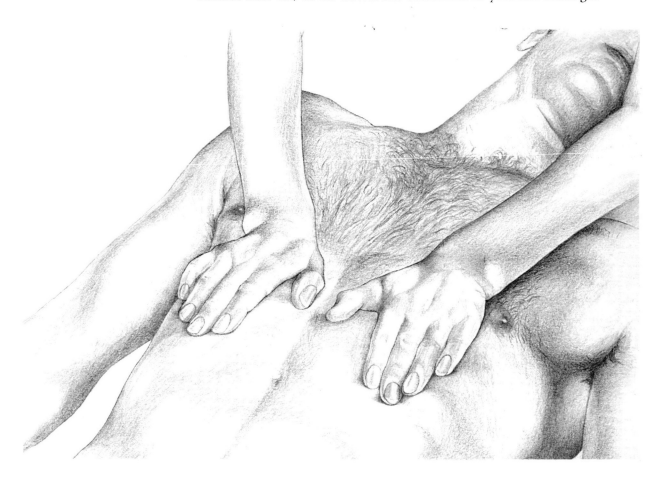

Then separate the hands, moving to your partner's sides and bring them over and down the hips until they touch the floor. Once they touch the floor, pull your hands slowly but firmly along the underneath of the torso in the direction of the head. Put your whole body into the pull until your hands reach the armpits and almost lift your partner off the floor.

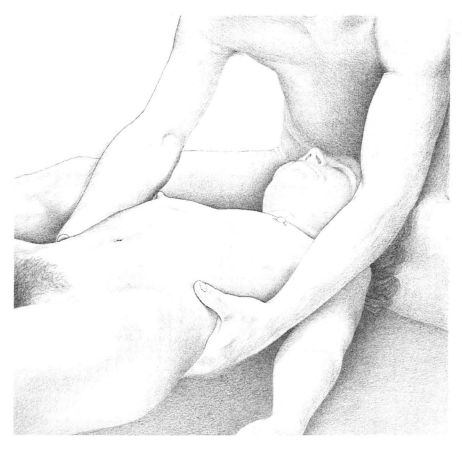

Pulling along the sides *Pull your hand slowly but firmly along the underneath of the torso in the direction of the head.*

Just before you actually touch the armpit, pull your hands (wrists first) up on the upper part of the chest. Swinging the fingertips round from the sides to the centre of the chest, glide the hands forward until they are back again into the starting position.

From here you can repeat the whole stroke without a break in motion. To ensure fluid movement, try to be steady and carry out the routine at an even pace. Remember to alter your hands to fit into your partner's shape so that you accommodate the stroke to their bumps and curves.

Variation One After pulling your arms up from the armpit, send them over and down the shoulders instead of swivelling them towards the middle of the chest. Continue without a pause, right under the shoulders, on to the topmost part of the back, inserting your fingers between their back and the floor. As soon as your fingers reach the spine (not actually *on* the spine), slide your hands up over the back, on to the shoulders and back on to the upper chest.

Variation Two   Slip your hands down the sides of the shoulders and on to the back as before. Once again, stop just short of the spine. This time, pull your hands lightly on to the back of the neck, palms uppermost, between the back of the head and the ground. Don't lift your hands off the ground, but very slowly pull the hands up towards you, allowing them to slip underneath the head and then pull away from underneath (at the top of the head) altogether. Return your hands to the starting position on the chest as quickly as possible.

These strokes can be repeated several times as the introduction to a chest and abdomen massage and can be used to link later strokes and even to finish the massage.

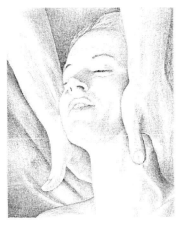

Variation II *Your hands pulling underneath the head, gently lift it off the ground with their movement, replacing it once they have passed on.*

FINGERTIP WORKOUT

Rest the fingertips of both hands lightly on your partner's upper chest. Pressing firmly, move the fingertips in tiny circles. Work systematically so that you have covered the whole of the upper chest. Do *not* include the breasts if your partner is a woman.

ABDOMEN ROTATION

Abdomen rotation *With the fingertips only, rotate the loose skin of the abdomen in small circles.*

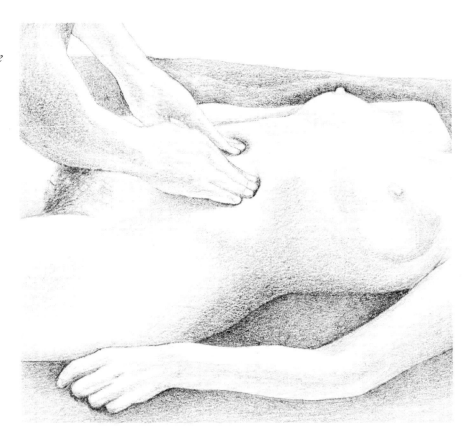

Cup your hands over the breasts and gently rotate the breasts as far as is comfortable in three complete circles. Move the breasts first towards each other and then for a second three circles away from each other.

BREAST STROKE

Start with the right side first. Kneeling to the right of your partner bring your right hand up, palms down, underneath the right-hand side of the right breast. When you reach the nipple move your thumb and first finger together – still with the palm covering the area – around the nipple. With the nipple as axis, rotate the right hand anti-clockwise, making a slight twisting of the nipple as the thumb and forefinger slide up and off the nipple.

BREAST AND NIPPLE KNEADING

While the right hand is rotating the left hand begins a similar movement from the opposite side, eventually to make a clockwise rotation. The complete stroke therefore is a continual movement of one hand after the other.

The success of this stroke depends largely on the amount of breast tissue there is to work with. To be blunt, it is much harder to carry out easily with someone flat-chested.

Repeat on the left side.

Think of the breast as a wheel with the nipple for axis once again and imagine 'spokes' radiating out from the axis. Both hands have finger and thumb positioned on the nipples. With a gentle squeeze, move the hands (resting on the ball of the finger and thumb) outwards, away from each other along the lines of the imaginary spokes. Repeat the movement following further along other imaginary spokes.

SPOKES STROKE

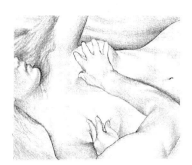

Kneeling at your partner's head, make both hands into fists. Rest them in the middle of the upper chest just below the collar bone with the backs of the upper parts of the fingers actually touching your partner. Pressing lightly, slide the fists apart to right and lift, over and across the upper chest to the armpit on each side. Repeat this movement until you have covered sections of the ribs, stopping at the stomach. Try to let individual knuckles slide between individual ribs. This should be a light stroke as a hard pressure will be uncomfortable. If your partner is female, do tiny versions of this between the breasts, but not actually on the breasts.

KNUCKLE NURTURE

PULLING

Move down your partner's right side to the right hip. Leaning over your partner, place both hands, palms down, on their left side with fingers pointing at the floor. Pull each hand up and off their torso, one after the other, keeping a continuous movement going and repeat this all the way up their side to the armpit, and then down again to the starting point.

Cross to their left side and repeat. When you pull at their body try to set a rocking motion going with their whole body, in time to your hands.

COLONIC MASSAGE

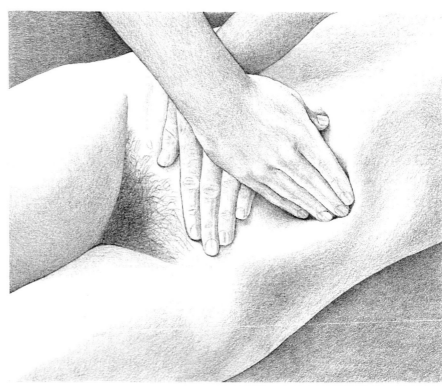

Colonic massage *Move the skin itself around and above the colon, working in a clockwise direction, from the lower right hand side of the abdomen, up and round to the left hand side.*

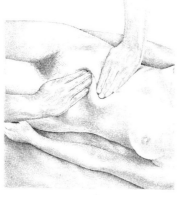

Using the fingers of the right hand in a duck's bill shape, massage the skin above the colon in a series of on-the-spot rotations, not actually moving the fingers on the skin but moving the skin itself around the above the colon. Start at the beginning of the colon on the left-hand side of the pelvis near to the hip bone, work your way up the line of the colon, along the top of the colon (just below waist level), then down the right-hand side of the abdomen. It doesn't matter if you aren't 100 per cent accurate about locating the colon – any continuous movement in this circular area will feel good.

KNEADING

Position yourself at your partner's right side, level with their waistline. Reaching across their body place both hands on their left side at the waist and gently knead the spare flesh there between finger and thumb, exactly as if you were kneading dough or pastry. Make sure that your hands move a little with each kneading movement so that a different part is covered each time. When you have kneaded as much as feels comfortable, move to the opposite side of your partner and repeat the stroke.

This is a dramatic stroke with which to finish. Kneel astride your partner's thighs and slide both hands, palms up, underneath your partner's back until your hands meet together underneath their spine. Lace your fingers together beneath the spine itself and lift the middle of your partner's body clear of the floor for a few seconds.

SPINAL LIFT

Spinal lift *Kneel astride your partner's thighs, lace your fingers together beneath the spine and lift for a few seconds. This is a dramatic stroke with which to finish.*

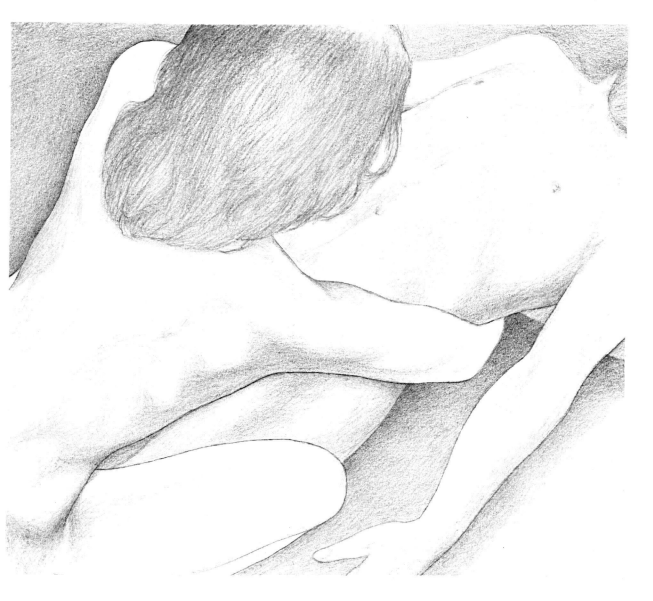

Repeat this lift two further times and as you let your hands down for the last time slide them out from under your partner and slide them up their waist until your fingers meet across their navel and slowly lift off.

The chest and abdomen massage is a continuation of our journey across the body. It is also a continuation of the way in which we learn about touch falling naturally between a back massage and some of the more erotic strokes which the next chapter includes. It acts as part of a continuation process in the *emotional* life of the two people who practise the strokes. Above all, it is a means of ensuring deep pleasure and relaxation.

For adults only – erotic massage

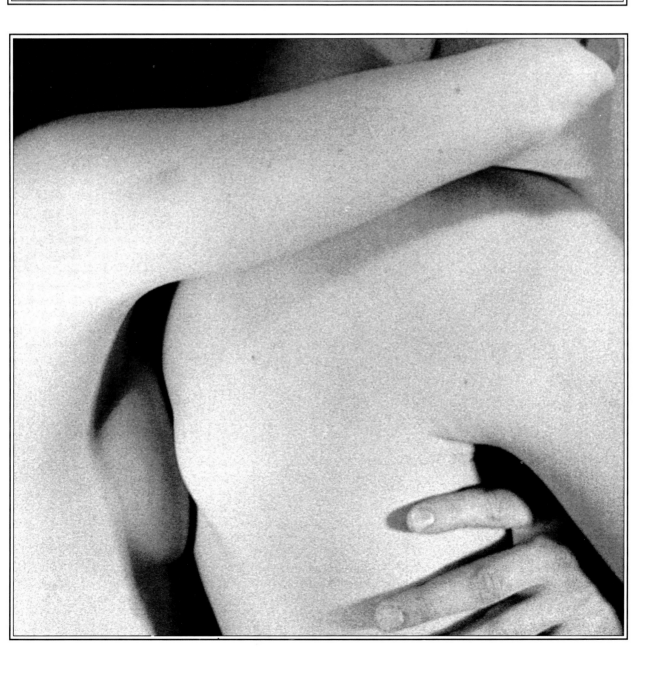

The touch described so far has been non-erotic, deliberately so, in order that the exercises are non-threatening and therefore acceptable to new friends and partners. This chapter sees a change. It is aimed at those who make the conscious decision that they want to take massage further. It is aimed at couples in long-term relationships and, although it may be used by friends, the friends need to possess a basic trust in each other.

The quality of touch

Most people think an erotic massage is one that is focused on the genitals. Indeed, there are specific massages for these areas, but an erotic massage takes in the whole body, for the greatest sex organ of all is the skin.

In view of the previous guidelines outlining the difference between a sensual massage and a sexual one, it may seem surprising (and confusing) to hear that all the body massages detailed so far, can be transformed into erotic ones. The difference lies in the quality of touch and the new realisation that the sexual element is something you both want. A basic similarity is retained, though, in the continuing framework of not working towards masturbation or intercourse and not expecting any kind of 'pay-off' in the shape of a climax or a voyeuristic 'buzz'.

Where previously you may have touched with a firm stroke, a lighter one will now bring *erotic* sensation to the surface. Where formerly you gained relaxation with deep massage, now you achieve stimulation at *fingertip level*. The most skilful part of this process is making the transition from sensual massage to deliberately erotic touch. The time to make the change arrives only with the realisation that *you both want to do it*. At no time should an erotic massage be carried out without the full and enthusiastic consent of both partners.

Neither should you ever allow what has started off as a sensual massage to change halfway through into an erotic one. If you make an agreement at the beginning of a massage you must stick to it, however much your feelings may alter. If you don't, the agreement is valueless and you will have shown you are a person not to be trusted. Since trust is the most basic ingredient of massage, keeping contracts is vital.

However it is also normal to learn from experience and if you are now feeling such pleasure in each other's company you want to go further, the time has come for discussion. Perhaps your partner only waits for a cue from you. If you are agreed erotic massage is for you, the *next* session, *not* the present one, can mark a new departure.

Crossing the sensual boundaries

If at any time in the session, either of you feels uncomfortable with what is happening, the agreement must be to stop. There is no point in enduring something which creates tension and discomfort – those are *not* the aims of good touch – but it is worth talking about the problem in order to resolve it.

One difficulty which commonly arises is fear that sexual arousal will get in the way of enjoyment: 'What will I look like?' 'How will I behave?' 'Will I make a fool of myself?' Naturally these anxieties need to be heard and reassurance given. It may help to know that men and women enjoying an erotic massage look much as they do during an ordinary sensual one. Just as they are receptive to full body massage, so are they open to a genital one. But since an erotic massage consists of touching the entire body and *not only the genitals*, this division won't actually exist.

'Suppose I get a climax?' Although a climax is not an aim it may, of course, happen by accident and it is important to feel all right about it. You might tell your partner that if this does happen it will be fine and you will be pleased for them. If you cannot offer this reassurance you are not ready for erotic massage. Skilful use of the energy sweep (see page 59), however, can ward off the likelihood of a climax and also allow the partner to get maximum prolonged skin sensation.

Readers may wonder at the logic of curtailing erotic pleasure by avoiding orgasm. The explanation is that erotic pleasure is not curtailed – it is allowed to take a different pathway. An erotic massage is a way of experiencing great sensual delight and is an alternative to orgasm, rather than a route to it.

These discussions are part of the transition. Meanwhile the basic agreements of no intercourse and no deliberate stimulation for the purpose of intercourse may also be established.

What about the couples where one partner decides that he or she just isn't ready for such a major change? Their decision must be respected, but the hesitant partner should be prepared for further discussion at a later date. The decision *not* to start also deserves analysis. What kind of feeling does erotic massage throw up? What fears are there? What might this say or show about the hesitant partner? Or about the relationship between both partners? Un-blocking fears and feelings through this process sometimes changes the decision.

Doing an erotic massage for the first time may bring to the surface anxieties about your ability as a masseur. The following is an excerpt from a personal account of first-time erotic massage. It illustrates these anxieties, but it also shows how quickly you can over come them.

I am a little scared in case my unsure touch should be an anti-climax after the mass of sensation he'd provoked between us, but he is pleased at the suggestion. He is glad I want to contribute too, that it isn't only a one-way happening. So he takes off his clothes and lies down before the fire and I go to work on him, occasionally receiving instructions. It is quite a trip to know that you are pleasing someone so much. And the more I tune in to him and the pleasures he is receiving, the more daring I feel. I dare concentrate on his erogenous zones; I massage his bottom with confidence. (It's quite daunting faced with a strange derrière to know just how intimate you can and ought to be . . .) His bottom turns out to be the most sensuous zone of his back. It

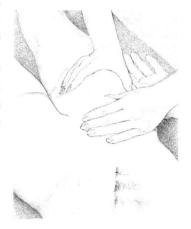

Buttock massage *Holding the top of the buttocks with one hand, run the flat of the other hand towards the first, across the surface of the buttock.*

gets so that I can touch him there, firmly, make my hands swim in circles, pull my fingertips deliberately over him. Whatever I do, he reacts violently and sexually.

It is almost frightening, observing the kind of power I momentarily hold over this man. And, learning from my own reactions, I know that the rest of his body is yearning to receive similar sensuality . . . If, after half an hour, I hadn't become so tired, I would happily have gone on for ever.

This description of a first ever erotic massage shows how ordinary massage strokes can be adapted to provide an erotic massage – for ordinary strokes these were. The only difference lay in how they were performed.

Erotic strokes – varying the quality

Using basic massage strokes, such as circling, swimming, etc., practise these at:
1. a deep, firm layer of pressure;
2. a relaxed pressure;
3. a fingertip layer.

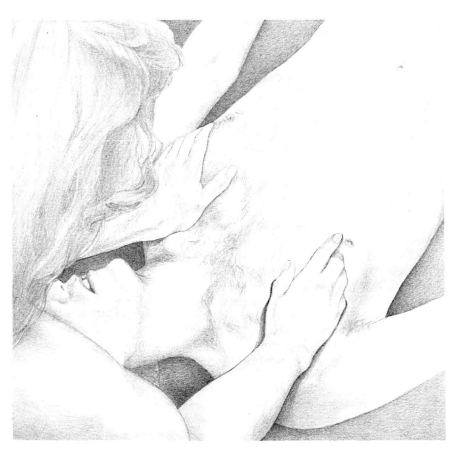

Circling nipples *With the forefinger slowly and deliberately circle around the nipples.*

1. Use the balls of the fingers, pressing hard;
2. pressing lightly.
3. Make sure the nails touch the surface of the skin.
4. Scratch the skin with the fingernails only.
5. Vary the scratching so that some is in circles;
6. some from side to side;
7. some up and down;
8. some are long strokes;
9. some are very short strokes.

1. The frivolous follicles stroke or hair massage (see page 16).
2. Slowly, with one finger, circle the inside of the ear, tracing its outline softly.
3. Put your mouth close to the ear and breathe softly on it.
4. Breathe on the neck.
5. Draw your fingernails gently down the inner arm.
6. Circle the nipples with a fingernail.
7. Softly pinch the nipple between finger and thumb.
8. Stroke down the sides of each breast.
9. Breathe on the nipples.
10. If you have long hair, sweep it slowly across your partner's abdomen.
11. Follow this up with light fingertip circling of the abdomen.
12. Run your fingertips up the inner thigh, stopping at the genitals.
13. Repeat but finish by brushing against the genitals.
14. Deep massage your partner's palms with yours.
15. Fingertip circle around the palm of the hands.
16. Exquisitely and slowly, pull a finger between each of the toes.

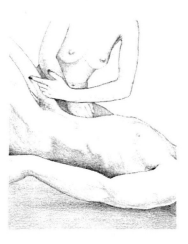

Fingertip massage *Vary your touch with fingertip strokes instead of deep pressure.*

Erotic massage for women

Peacock feathers, fur gloves, a warm bath, a hot towel and an erotic massage that lasts for hours sound like elements from some kind of fantastic dream. These were all ingredients of a wonderful treat I received at the hands of Ray Stubbs in San Francisco's Institute for the Advanced Study of Human Sexuality.

Returning to England I hastened to pass my good fortune on to others. Here is what I wrote.

It is important to understand that maximum body enjoyment is the result of maximum body relaxation and trust. A lovely way to begin the massage is to have a warm bath together. Make a point of using sweet-smelling bath oils, and to soap each other as lovingly and carefully as you would a baby. When your partner is ready to step out of the bath, be careful to ensure that there are hot fluffy towels waiting to cradle her and that you pamper your friend by drying her and holding her close to you.

Hot towels *Make sure there are hot, fluffy towels waiting to cradle your partner after the bath.*

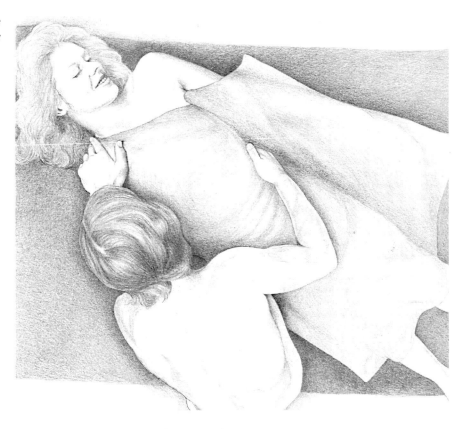

The very best erotic massage starts with a full body massage (see previous chapters on back massage and chest and abdomen massage), so that you have opportunities to discover the sensitive parts of her body other than her genital area. Additional strokes to include are brushing her lightly all over with a feather (before you coat her with warm oil) and following this up with stroking her all over with either a fur glove or if you don't have one, a piece of soft fur.

Once you have worked your way through the whole body massage which as in previous massages should be carried out naked in a warm room with low lights, you are ready for the genital strokes.

The emphasis throughout is on going SLOWLY. Do everything in slow motion; take a long, long time over giving your partner her pleasure. A good erotic massage takes at least an hour. Mine, in San Francisco, took a dizzying three hours.

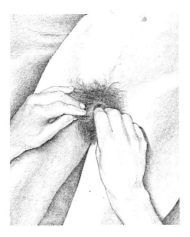

Gentle hair tease

Very slowly and very gently tug tiny clumps of pubic hair one after the other.

Don't think twice about it and don't question this instruction – just begin by pulling her pubic hairs, almost one by one, very gently and very slowly. Work your way from the top of the pubic triangle, right down to the hairs on each side of the labia between her legs. Take a long unhurried time over this and I promise you'll be appreciated.

Take a bottle of warm oil in your left hand. Slowly and carefully pour a little of it over your right hand shaped with the fingers pointing downwards and together, looking a little like a duck's bill. The object of this is to allow the oil to seep slowly through your fingers and down your fingertips so that it runs on to and down her genitals. It feels, to the woman, like a safe flood of warmth. (Now you can understand the necessity for the oil to be gently heated. Flooding with cold oil is a nasty experience. The best way to heat the oil is to float the bottle in the bath at the start of an evening.)

Drowning

Separate the outer lips of the vagina from the inner and, with both hands on one outer lip, gently pull and let go, pull and let go, in a rhythmic pattern, starting at the very end of the lip away from the clitoris and working up the lip towards the clitoris. A good analogy for this movement is the kind of lip pulling children sometimes do on their mouth to make funny little flapping sounds.

Pulling

You could pull the lip perhaps half a dozen times or more on your journey up. Then repeat, very gently, on the other side. Then repeat with a hand on each lip at the same time. Do the same with the inner lips, starting with first one, then the other, then both at the same time.

You may need to separate the inner lips when you begin, but it is quite likely that your partner will have become aroused and if this is the case her labia will have swelled a little and naturally separated. The inner lips usually meet over the clitoris forming the clitoral hood and when you reach the clitoral end make sure that you continue the pulling-then-letting-go gently over the clitoral hood as well.

With the forefinger, carefully and sensitively run your finger around and around the clitoris, never touching the top, simply circling and circling. After a dozen or so circles change the stroke to rubbing lightly up and down on the left side of the clitoris a dozen times, then on the right side of the clitoris a dozen times. Still with the forefingers, rub backwards and forwards immediately below the clitoris a dozen times and then from the clitoris down to the opening of the vagina and back, also a dozen times.Men tend to think women prefer clitoral stimulation to be firm and direct, but this isn't always the case.

Circling

The lemon squeezer, the corkscrew, the hand over hand – they sound a little like American cocktails, don't they? They are from America, yes, but drinks, no, though cocktails may be an apter description than I'd originally realised. These are the names given to some of the strokes given in Ray Stubbs' class of erotic massage for

Erotic massage for men

men. As with the women's massage an all-over body massage enhances anything that comes after it. It's up to you if you decide to make short cuts but be warned. The build-up of erotic sensation will be much less intense and therefore less enjoyable.

As with the previous massage the emphasis is on being SLOW. Warmth and romantic lighting all help set the scene (see page 29).

Coating your warmed hands with warmed oil, gently but firmly stroke it into your partner's genitals and that includes his penis, testicles and perineum.

When you are sure that he is sufficiently slippery to cut out any possibility of catching and pulling unpleasantly at his skin (hairy men need more oil than others), you begin with the first basic strokes.

The count-down

With the right hand gripping the top of the penis and the left underneath the testicles (fingers on the perineum pointing towards the anus), run the right hand down the penis, at the same time sliding the left hand up the underside of the testicles. You are thus bringing both hands towards and past each other. This is the first stroke of the count-down.

The second stroke begins with the right hand gripping the base of the penis while the left hand (fingers pointing downward, with the palm placed on the top of the testicles) is as near to the penis base as possible. Slowly and gently run the right hand, still gripping the penis, up the shaft, and at the same time push the left hand down and over the testicles, so that you are effectively reversing the first stroke.

The count-down then consists of ten times the first stroke, then ten times the second, then nine times the first stroke and nine times the second, then eight times the first stroke and eight times the second and so on down to one of each. Which brings us to . . .

The corkscrew

Grip the penis gently with both hands and slide both hands around the penis in opposite directions at the same time as though you were trying to twist the penis in half . . . . ! And then back again. I hardly need emphasise that you do this GENTLY. Repeat ten times.

The lemon squeezer

Gripping the penis about half way up with the left hand, rub your cupped right hand over and around the top of the penis head, as if you were juicing a lemon. Repeat 10 times clockwise and then ten times anti-clockwise.

Hand over hand

Fairly quickly, place first one cupped hand over the head of the penis (changing from cupping as it leaves the head to gripping the circumference till it reaches the base), then the other cupped hand which repeats the performance. Keep moving hand over hand in this way. The object is never to let the head of the penis be uncovered, rather like the childish game of 'hand over hand'.

These then are the basic strokes. Once you have gone through the whole collection you may use them in whichever order you prefer. Obviously the first time you practise with your partner, it's a good idea to check what kind of pressure he prefers.

I emphasise again that it is better to include a whole body massage with a genital massage. There is discernable difference in quality.

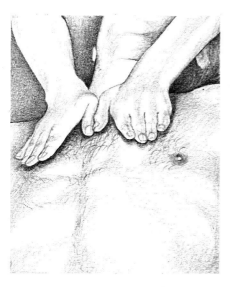

Energy sweep *Brush away feelings of excess energy by skimming your partners body with the flat of your hand held above the skin,* not actually touching it. *Sweep the energy away and out of the air above the hands, feet and head.*

The energy sweep

If either man or woman becomes very stimulated by the genital massage but does not climax, a good way of defusing their sexual energy is as follows. With hands held flat, about an inch above the body (like a hovercraft) sweep the energy that the body is radiating out of the hands, the feet and the head. You don't need to actually touch your partner to do this. Just skim your hands above their body as I have described. A surprising feeling of completion is reported by the receivers once their massage has been terminated in this way.

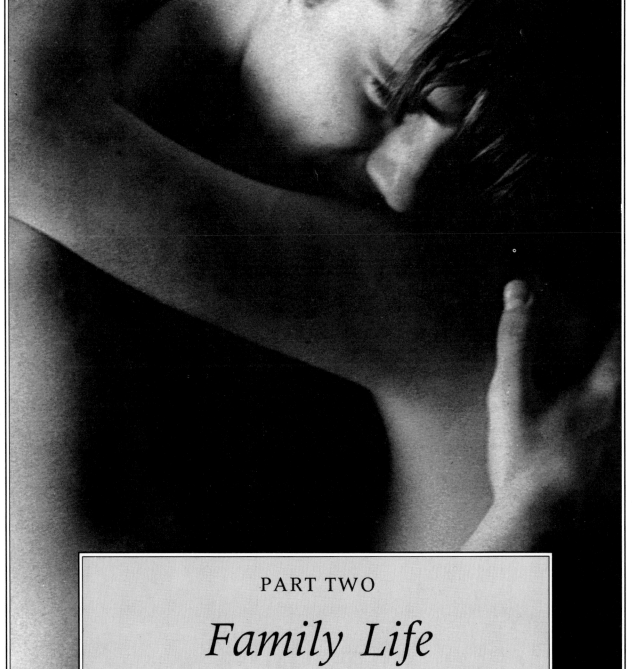

PART TWO

Family Life

Touch as sex therapy

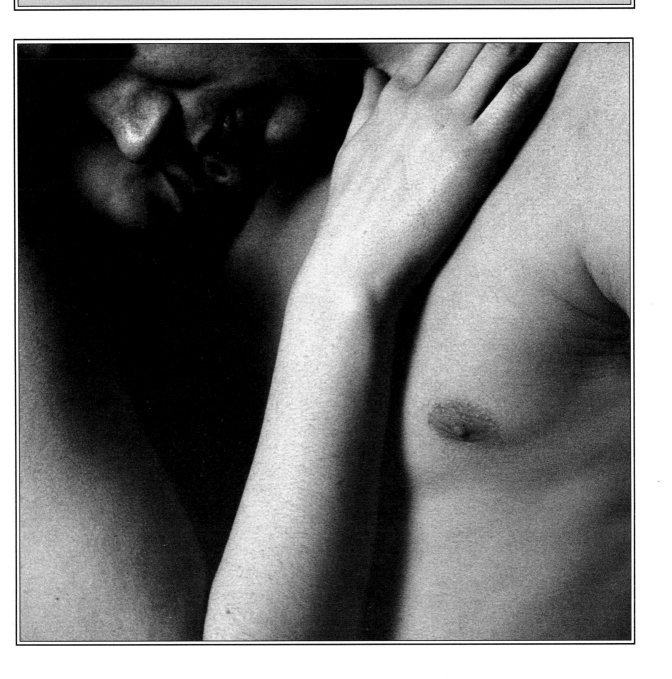

'And they lived happily ever after' – the phrase assumes a lot. It assumes that a couple are compatible in the way they share their life, make love, treat their friends and family and combine interests.

Yet hazards crop up which make marriage or long-term relationships an emotional obstacle course. Fatigue, stress, boredom, children, ill-health, all contribute to sabotage nuptial bliss. Nevertheless, some hardy couples survive, apparently using superhuman strength to do so. What this strength consists of is a matter of speculation.

I suspect the secret to remaining happy ever after lies in a sense of continuity. If you possess an ability to view the ups and downs of marriage as a long-term pattern, rather than opt out at the first major row, you retain a greater chance of surviving the 'downs'. People who thus perceive the cyclic shape that marital life takes on are frequently aided by the belief that a bond exists between them and their partner. When times are bad, the memory of that bond encourages endurance. The bond itself can be as nebulous as lovemaking when all else has failed or as tough as an unshakeable mutual belief. It doesn't really matter what it is, as long as such a tie is there, serving as a bedrock for the rest of the relationship.

Touch plays a big part in long-term bonding. Most happy marriages report a high ratio of touch, cuddles and hugs. And most happy marriages include sex in the touch list. But sometimes sexual touch goes sour or is misinterpreted as sexual pressure. When this happens it is often the result of a common confusion made between sexuality and love. There are thousands of people who think that having sex means showing love and this is complicated by the fact that sex can be greatly enhanced by loving feelings.

Very often the partner who is asking for a lot of sex is really asking for a lot of love. If the spouse can't cope with their greedy demands (for sex) and rejects them, it can seem as if they are also denying love (when all they are really asking for is a 'breather'). Sometimes substituting extra cuddles *without* sex, succeeds in driving home the message that the needy partner *is* loved; it doesn't have to be 'proved' by a repetitive act of sex. In order to accept this change in ideals however partners need to rethink their ideas about marital touch. Sex therapy, through special touch exercises, helps to do this. (Psychological theory has it incidentally that many prostitutes are mistakenly seeking love and affection through the repeated sex act.)

Sometimes the problem veers off in a different direction. The desire for sex disappears altogether. Or a partner wants to enjoy sex but finds it keeps going wrong. Disentangling the reasons taxes sexologists still, but there is basic agreement about some of the more common sexual problems.

Romantic myth

It doesn't help when one romantic myth maintains that if a couple gets on well enough they will be able to solve any problem, thanks to their ability 'to talk it through'. Highly intelligent people still believe this today. While it is undoubtedly true that good communication is a vital ingredient of what makes a relationship work, if the sexual element is not right it can insidiously corrode a couple's feelings so that the most loving pair cool off each other. Clinical evidence indicates that between 10 to 20 per cent of young couples are sexually unsuccessful during the first years of marriage and that if the problem continues the marriage is more than likely to become unhappy.

When sexuality deserts a marriage the cause can often be found in the sufferers past. Perhaps they associate marriage with family, therefore sexual relations suddenly become incestuous. Perhaps an element of competition creeps in with disastrous results. Perhaps a marriage partner is seen as pure and therefore unexciting. Sex therapists these days use a combination of psychotherapy and touch exercise to help such unhappy couples.

There is of course a range of people whose sex life chunters on very adequately over the years but remains low key. They don't want to swing from a chandelier, but they would like to light a new candle. By using touch to think about sensuality differently they can achieve this, though sometimes they need to go through a phase of *un*-learning in order to do so.

How sexual response is learned

We learn about our own sexuality by accident. Most of us (but not all) discover our genitals when very young and associate good sensation with them. Boys, for obvious reasons, discover their genitals with more ease than girls and generally become skilled in pleasuring themselves at an early age. By the time they are teenagers, they have usually conditioned themselves to think of sexuality as an 'external' genital event.

Girls, on the other hand, are often actively *dis*couraged from finding their genitals when young and therefore don't associate sexuality with a particular behaviour or area of the body. Sexual familiarity for women often comes later, during the teens, when romantic fiction may be the path to self-pleasure. Most (but not all) women discover their sexual response by their 20s – frequently by a route of passionate fantasy and personal 'exploration'. As a result of this 'route' women therefore tend to 'internalise' sex feelings more than men.

When eventually man and woman meet, these opposite paths to self-discovery mean they come to mutual sex from very different viewpoints. The majority of couples learn from each other, combining passionate thoughts with practical stimulation. Not everybody, however, is skilled at tuning into other people's thought processes. If they can't understand their partner's sexual pattern, they may need help, which is where touch therapy comes in.

Why touch therapy?

The value of touch therapy is that it takes you back to the early days of mutual exploration, days when you were only finding out about each other and not expected to produce orgasms at the drop of a hat. Once upon a time couples enjoyed heavy petting, an excellent method of learning each other's response. Sex therapy takes you back to the days of petting.

'Communication' however is not forgotten. As you re-learn how to caress your partner's body you are encouraged to share his/her feelings and reactions while he/she is asked to voice them. Ideally you are learning to trust each other while growing comfortable with sex. With any luck, you will also be having fun.

The routine which follows is designed to enhance the lovemaking of people who already enjoy good sex, but it can, in addition, be used by people with sexual dysfunction. Further exercises follow the enhancement routine for the benefit of people with premature ejaculation, impotence or inability (on the part of the woman) to experience orgasm.

Sexual enhancement routine

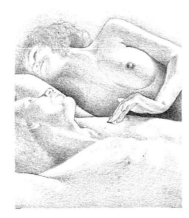

+3−3 A touch game to measure erotic reaction. Each stroke covers only two inches of the skin.

PHASE ONE   Over a period of two or three weeks

1. The Foot Bath (see page 17)
2. The Hair Sweep (see page 14)
3. Spoons (see page 27)
4. Mirror on the wall (see page 27)
5. Hand play (see page 27)
6. Cuddling (see page 27)
7. Finger tipping (see page 27)
8. Bathing together. Rub and soap each other caressingly in the warm water.
9. Plus Three–Minus Three (see page 28)

PHASE TWO   Over two days

1. *His genitals*   He lies back while she looks carefully at his genitals, holding him and moving him so that she can examine every aspect. When this is done, a detailed repetition follows of Plus Three–Minus Three on his genitals with discussion of how it feels.
2. *Her genitals*   Follow the same routine as for his genitals. The purpose of these two exercises is to de-mystify the genitals and to let couples become familiar with parts of the body which previously made them feel shy. Plus Three–Minus Three on the genitals provides useful information about reaction to touch and often comes up with surprises. (For example, most people think that a woman's vagina has no sensation, but there are certain areas which respond with sensitivity.)

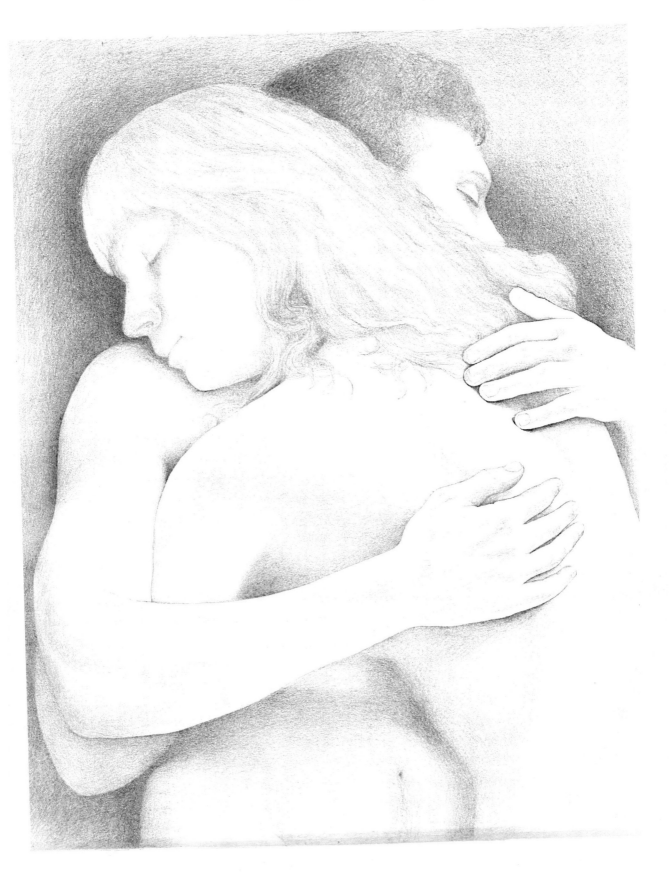

PHASE THREE   Two or three hourly sessions a week in a warm room where you will be private

1. You agree not to have intercourse. (This removes any performance demands.)
2. For half an hour each one of you massages the other. The one being massaged tells the other exactly how it feels to be touched in every part of the body – except the genitals which you may not touch at this stage – and describes in turn how he/she would like to be touched. You are just trying to give and receive pleasure at this stage.

PHASE FOUR   Two or three hourly sessions a week as before

1. You agree not to have intercourse.
2. Continue with the massages, but this time include the genitals. The purpose is to provide information about response to touch and to give good sensual feeling. The man should explain how he likes to be touched on his penis and the woman how she likes to be touched on, at or near the vagina and clitoris. You *are* trying to give pleasure, but you are *not* trying to give an orgasm.

From here on touch therapy diversifies to suit the special problems of the individual couple. If however you are using the touch enhancement programme you may follow the next phases (Five and Six designed specifically for men with impotence and described below), but may readapt them to suit your circumstances. More attention can be paid to the needs of the female partner's pleasure and although the stop/start methods used in the impotence exercises won't be strictly necessary they are very good for helping build up intense sexual feeling rather than letting it dissipate in an early climax.

Impotence

There are several types of impotence. Lifelong impotence is when a man has never had an erection or orgasm in his life, either with or without a partner. Men with this condition should seek specific medical advice since touch therapy will not be of much help.

A second type is when a man may never have been potent with a woman, but has been quite capable of a good sexual response when masturbating and during sleep. Medical advice should be sought but some touch therapy may be of assistance here.

A third category is usually defined as the case of a man who has been previously potent with a woman, but is no longer so. And a 'sub-division' of this sort of selective impotence is the case of the man who is potent only with particular types of women. Both types should find touch therapy of help. The majority of cases fall into this third category.

Touch therapy for impotence follows the sexual enhancement

programme from Phase One through to Phase Four as described earlier, then progresses to Phase Five.

PHASE FIVE   Two or three times over the period of a week

The emphasis for the moment is on pleasure for the male. If the female partner also wants to be pleasured a separate agreement must be made for her at some other time.
1. You agree that intercourse is banned.
2. You continue Phase Four. The man may get an erection at this stage. If he does, you should tease and cease stimulation in that area. When the erection has subsided then the women should provoke it again. Once you can do this together, the man will regain confidence from knowing that he can regain an erection after he has lost it.

PHASE SIX   Two or three times a week over the period of a fortnight

1. The intercourse ban is lifted.
2. The woman teases the man to erection by straddling him while he is lying on his back. She must not try and climax at this point, but simply put his penis inside her vagina. If the erection goes down she lifts herself away and teases the erection back (as in Phase Five). Once he is able to maintain his erection, she begins to thrust gently while he keeps still. When he knows he can cope with this, it is his turn to thrust from beneath while the woman keeps still. This is meant to be gentle and aimless. Climax is not a goal – the goal is good feeling.

As the routine is followed the man will be able to last out longer and longer with the thrusting until he has managed it for fifteen minutes. He can now be said to have overcome his impotence. As the couple grows familiar with the procedure it will cease feeling like an exercise and become more like making love. If, at any stage, the man feels pressurised or panic-stricken, it means he is going too fast. In this case you should retreat to an earlier stage and learn to feel comfortable with that before advancing again.

If there are difficulties in following the touch therapy routine successfully, there may be hidden resentments and unexpressed anger getting in the way of success. If it is difficult to resolve these, this is a sensible stage at which to enlist the help of a marriage counsellor or sex therapist. Touch therapy can still be followed but within the context of counselling. (For detailed information about the condition of impotence see *The Thinking Woman's Guide to Sex* by Anne Hooper.)

Premature ejaculation

A premature ejaculator is defined as someone who would like to last longer sexually but for a number of reasons cannot do so. He may have been conditioned by early experiences of sex (in hurried situations, perhaps) to come quickly. Having learned this pattern he cannot escape it. Alternatively he may be extremely tense and nervous about sex generally and expresses this tension by ejaculating too soon. Both these types of premature ejaculator will find touch therapy of assistance.

There is also a third sort where the man expresses resentment against a partner by ejaculating prematurely, in a subconscious attempt to punish her. This is a relationship problem rather than a sexual one and will benefit more from counselling than touch therapy.

The premature ejaculator needs to learn to distinguish between arousal and the 'point of no return' just prior to climax. Touch therapy encourages him to get to know his own sexual response well in order to do this before moving on to partner-assisted work. It is therefore structured in two halves: in the first, the male works by himself; in the second he is joined by his partner. All work is done for the benefit of the male alone. If the female also needs sexual pleasure then a separate agreement should be made between them to arrange time to spend on her.

The therapy is usually practised over a matter of weeks. It is important that before continuing to a further stage the preceeding one is satisfactorily completed.

Premature ejaculation therapy

For him alone

1. Masturbate with a dry hand until you can last fifteen minutes.
2. Masturbate with a lubricated hand until you can last fifteen minutes.

For you both

3. She masturbates him with a dry hand until he can last fifteen minutes.
4. She masturbates him with a lubricated hand until he can last for fifteen minutes.
5. The male lies on his back with the woman astride. His penis is contained in her vagina, moving only the minimum needed to retain erection until he can last this way for fifteen minutes.
6. She sits astride him and thrusts gently while he remains on his back immobile, until he can last for fifteen minutes.
7. She sits astride him while *he* thrusts gently until he can last for fifteen minutes.
8. She sits astride him and both thrust until he can last for fifteen minutes.

If, at any stage of this therapy either of you need help in preventing ejaculation, there are two methods of doing this.

When the man recognises the warning signs of ejaculation he must learn to tell you. At this point the woman stops all stimulation and prevents ejaculation by applying the squeeze. This consists of holding the head of the penis between fingers and thumb. The thumb is on the fraenulum of the penis between the glans and the second and third fingers are on either side of the coronal ridge. (When a man looks down at his penis the coronal ridge is topside and the fraenulum bottomside of his penis.)

THE SQUEEZE TECHNIQUE

The woman then squeezes hard (when the penis is erect squeezing causes little discomfort). A good way of learning how strong a squeeze is appropriate is to ask your partner to squeeze over your fingers, so that you understand just what pressure is suitable. After one squeeze the woman rests for a few seconds then applies it again. After two or three squeezes, each time with a pause between, the ejaculation will subside. So too may the erection. This then is the cue for further stimulation of the sort so far practised.

The squeeze needs to be practised several times a day for a few days until both partners feel comfortable that it works and that he is capable of regaining his erection afterwards. It is best to practise this during masturbation rather than intercourse. When the use of two or three squeezes has prolonged intercourse for about fifteen minutes the method can safely be said to be completed.

The Beautrais Manoevure is a squeeze alternative with the advantage that the man can apply it to himself. At the 'point of no return' the testicles rise, preparatory to ejaculation and the spermatic cord tenses. If, when this state is reached, a man reaches round behind himself and gently pulls the testicles down he will defer and delay orgasm.

THE BEAUTRAIS MANOEUVRE

Of course there may be hidden reasons why premature ejaculation therapy doesn't work. If you get 'stuck' at one stage and can't seem to get any further this indicates some outside help is needed in the shape of a sex therapist or counsellor.

Only a minority of women are unable to experience orgasm at all. Figures from the Hite Report, based on a survey of 3,000 women in the state of New York, showed that 82 per cent of female respondents enjoyed orgasm regularly through masturbation, but only 30 per cent managed it through intercourse.

Inability on the part of the woman to experience orgasm

Of the remaining 18 per cent who do not enjoy orgasm, clinical evidence shows that about 8 or 10 per cent are capable of learning how to experience orgasm while, so far, the last 10 per cent or so are not. However, recent sexological research tells us that there are likely to be organic reasons why this stubborn percentage fails to respond to touch therapy. If this seems to apply to you the best move is to seek referral to the most highly rated sexological specialist available, since the strides that are being made in hormone therapy and under-standing of nerve damage are growing from year to year.

Learning to experience orgasm through group work and 'self-pleasuring' homework is widely thought to be the most successful method of learning. However there are many couples who would like to work on the problem together and indeed many who like to experience their orgasms together. What follows here therefore is a combined touch therapy where work done by the individual woman can be combined with work done together as a couple.

Individual 'self-pleasuring' therapy

1. As Day One in the three-day self-massage routine (see page 41).
2. As Day Two in the three-day self-massage routine (see page 42).
3. As Day Three, Part 1 in the three-day self-massage (see page 42).
4. Explore the genitals more fully, not aiming at orgasm but simply re-awakening good feelings.
5. Repeat the previous step taking it further and build on the feelings of excitement. If you feel yourself approaching climax continue the stimulation in order to find out what happens. It is worth experimenting with many types of stimulation to discover what best suits you. Some women prefer a very light touch, some a hard pressure. Some prefer smooth up and down movements on one particular side of the clitoris, others prefer to roughly include both clitoris and vagina. Undoubtedly though the clitoris reacts most strongly to stimulation and it is important to note that if orgasm begins stimulation *continues to be needed* until the orgasm has eventually finished. If you stop the stimulation when orgasm is reached, unlike the male who *will* continue with ejaculation, the woman's sensations simply go away and the orgasm is incomplete.
6. If the 'self-pleasuring' provides good sensations, but not orgasm then using a vibrator, in the same way as you might fingers will give a faster and stronger stimulation. For the small percentage of women who need something extra to bring their climax 'over the top', a vibrator is often an excellent aid. Some women find that by learning to climax with a vibrator they can graduate from that to fingers and eventually, fingers combined with intercourse.

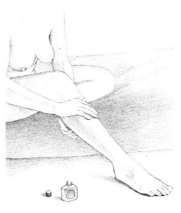

Self-pleasuring *Slowly and sensuously oil or cream the skin.*

The Kegels, named after their inventor, Dr Arnold Kegel, are routine exercise often recommended to women before and after childbirth in order to improve the muscle tone of the pelvic floor and vagina. Many women have found that after about six weeks of practising the exercise they experience increased pleasure during sexual intercourse. Exercising these muscles increases sensitivity in the vaginal area and also helps reduce accidental urination. Men can carry out similar 'contract-and-relax' exercises on the penis, building up muscle tone there and enabling them to enjoy a stronger orgasm.

The first step is to find PC (pubococcygeal) muscle. Do this by trying to stop and start the flow of your urine next time you go to the lavatory. The muscle that you use to slow down and stop the flow is the PC muscle. Practise stopping and starting the flow several times in order to get used to it.

The main Kegel exercise consists of squeezing the PC muscle for three seconds, then relaxing it for three seconds, then repeating this. Try doing this ten times, on three separate occasions every day. The beauty of the Kegels is that you can do them anywhere, while standing at the bus stop or doing the gardening.

Some couples prefer to work on the woman's sex problem together, each learning from the other. A similar self-pleasuring routine is followed, only for single bath, read double bath, and for self-touching read partner-touching. There is an agreement that there should be no intercourse and the couple (as in the impotence routine) learns to exchange information about giving and receiving sensual touch.

When the genital touch stage is reached, the routine alters and is as follows.

He leans back against the pillows in a sitting position while she leans against him. She is seated between his legs, with her back resting against his chest. From this vantage point he is able to hold her affectionately with one hand while placing the other between her legs. She places her own hand lightly over his so that she can signal to him manually to vary his touch.

He begins to explore her genitals by stroking the areas around them first, the insides of her thigh, above the pubis, in the creases between legs and abdomen before moving on to the perineum and labia. Aided by the feedback of her controlling hand, he slowly and sensuously moves towards the clitoris.

Rather than use hard, direct pressure on the clitoris he learns to work around it. Light up-and-down movements first on one side then the other, side-to-side movements either above or below the clitoris, fingertip twirling with a minute pressure on the top of the clitoris, are all suggested.

As in an ordinary massage, touch is enhanced by using some kind of lubricant. Natural vaginal juices are the obvious substance to fall easily to hand, but if this doesn't seem enough, massage oil can also be included.

The aim of these 'controlled 'sessions is to allow the male to discover his partner's erotic areas and to form a kind of erotic map through increasing familiarity with her response. As she can control the hand movements there need be no fear he will do something unacceptable and because there is no pressure to have a climax this need not surface as an anxiety.

The genital exercise is carried out three or four times so that the couple learns more and more about what turns her on. It is possible the woman will climax as a result of these 'explorations'. If she does, this is fine, a useful indication the method is working. If she doesn't, this is also valuable information and may indicate that continued practise incorporating a vibrator in the routine is appropriate.

If one member of the couple persistently finds difficulty in carrying out the routine or even seems to be deliberately sabotaging it at times, then extra help in the shape of a therapist is called for.

Massage for Parents-to-be

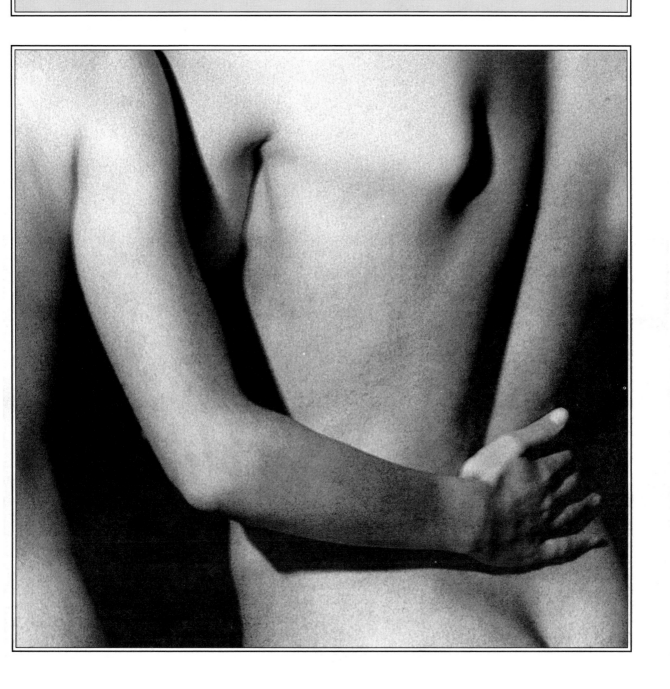

The value of touch in pregnancy

Mothers who have had a very recent experience of appropriate and meaningful bodily touch from a ministering person, as during labour, delivery, or the post-partum period, use their own hands more effectively. This is true of both . . . first-time mothers and . . . mothers who have had more than one child. Conversely, if the mother's most recent experiences of contact in relation to her own body have been of a remote and impersonal nature, she seems to stay longer at this stage in her own activities with the baby.

R. Rubin, 'Maternal touch', *Nursing Outlook*, 1963

If ever there was validation of the desirability for regular loving touch between a man and his pregnant partner, this is it. The addition of nurturing (in the shape of touch) to an expectant mother produces a genuine sense of well-being. It also, and more practically, offers her first-hand knowledge of the oldest method under the sun for pacifying little babies.

This is not the only reason for a man and woman to keep in touch on a physical level during pregnancy. The arrival of a first baby makes a massive change in the way the parents must live. Their entire lifestyle alters, creating new responsibilities and dependencies. The mother has to deal with a change of identity, loss of work, work contacts and friends, loss of intellectual stimuli, loss of sleep, the possibility, in the early days, of a body traumatised from the labour, physical exhaustion from breast feeding, unaccustomed stress from running around looking after a demanding baby and an urgent need to develop a brand-new set of friends with the same altered interests she is rapidly acquiring. In terms of shock to the system, her life, at this point, is one huge trauma. That most women survive pays tribute to their resilience.

The father, on the other hand, while not experiencing the same changes, is nevertheless subjected to them through his relationship with his partner; he is meeting and dealing with this changed person every day. And of course fathers have their own apprehensions and expectations of what it is to be a father, not to mention added financial pressures. Male needs during pregnancy have traditionally been unappreciated and one of the reasons male reactions *after* the birth are often distant and inappropriate is because they too need support and encouragement at this time, but are rarely offered it.

This is where massage during pregnancy can play a vital role. In order for the mother-to-be to feel happy and cared for, powerful doses of loving touch are required. One way of doing this is for her partner to give her aching body a gentle and caring massage at the end of the day. In order to allow him to do a great job of nurturing, the father-to-be needs some pay-off too. An occasional massage for *him* is one way of stiffling any niggling thoughts of 'she's awfully wrapped up in herself and doesn't seem to care much about me'.

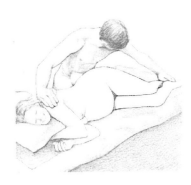

Comfortable Position *As the baby grows the mother-to-be prefers lying on her side so that her abdomen receives support. Massage along her side starting with your forearms resting on her waist, slowly separate the arms travelling in opposite directions till you end by lifting your arms off her, when they have reached as far as you can stretch.*

However, by finding the time to massage his partner's body, a man may also get pleasure himself. The fingertips are highly erotogenic. If you close your eyes while giving a massage and tune into the sensations in your own hands, you are in effect, massaging yourself. There is reward therefore in the attention a pregnant dad hands out to a pregnant mum.

It is hard for a man to understand the emotional, physical and mental changes a woman undergoes during pregnancy. The baby takes shape within a woman both literally and figuratively. Giving the father-to-be the opportunity to share in this process is therefore invaluable for the quality of the relationship of all three after the birth. And what better way for a father to get close to his partner *and* child than to massage them? As he sensitively kneads and caresses his partner's skin (incidentally increasing the blood supply to its surface) he can actually feel his child's reactions. If he is able to work out which way round his child is lying, he will recognise the movements of kicking and stretching – movements that *he* is responsible for stimulating.

There is a popular theory that tension affects babies 'in utero', producing chemical changes within their bodies. Following the same line of reasoning, it is possible to believe that the mother's pleasure and relaxation will also make an impact on the foetus bathing the unborn in pleasure and leaving him feeling as joyous and sensual as mum on the outside. Her massage might be the beginning of creating a happy and sensuous little person.

Physiological changes during pregnancy

The growing baby makes the most obvious change in a pregnant woman's body in her abdomen but there are many others happening alongside. The skin itself retains fluid more than when not-pregnant and the breasts in particular swell with extra fluid at a very early stage of pregnancy, becoming super sensitive to touch. One of the results of this extra fluid retention is a heightened level of sexual tension (not just during love-making but all the time!) This is why some women's sex lives improve dramatically during pregnancy.

However, muscular tension also increases from the sheer strain of carrying around those 20 odd extra pounds day and night, making it harder for women in the later stages of pregnancy to relax totally. The ideal state for the pregnant woman would be of course to have plenty of regular but gentle exercise, plenty of rest and plenty of sex. The reality is that most women don't get the time. They probably have to work, or to look after other children. If the other children are young, the mothers probably never get a chance to stop. This results in some very restless women, unable to sleep because they have been too exhausted to cope with the physical demands of intercourse but too 'strung up' from sexual tension in order to 'nod off'. Massage is a powerful tool for relaxation here.

Pregnancy massage

The altered state of the body during pregnancy means that there are some areas which would be best omitted from a massage. It is safe to say that the breasts are one area where it would be wise to go very carefully and ask for guidance. The 'bump' itself might feel uncomfortable with deep pressure strokes but might react with delight to fingertip massage. Deep pressure strokes or anything that involves leaning or putting the weight on to the partner's body should, for safety's sake, be avoided during pregnancy.

If the massager feels uncertain about where to touch it is sensible to carry out a pregnancy version of Plus Three–Minus Three (see page 28). But if you go carefully and ask for reactions continually, you should be able to avoid causing discomfort.

Most of the strokes of ordinary massage are suitable for pregnant women (provided as previously stated they do not depend on weight or pressure), but there are a few which are *specially* suitable to the pregnant body.

Positions

As her abdomen grows bigger, the pregnant mother will need to find her own most comfortable position in which to lie for a massage. Some like to lie on their sides with their stomach resting on the ground. In later pregnancy it may be wise to arrange cushions underneath the 'bump' to help support it and to lie on a mattress.

Pregnancy massage *As the baby grows the mother-to-be prefers lying on her side so that her abdomen receives support.*

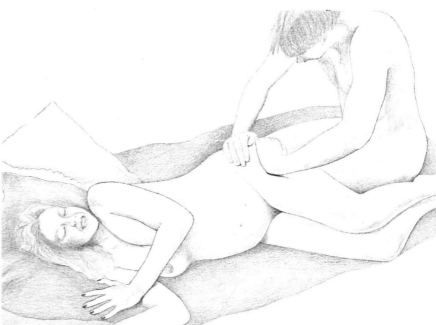

If during the later stages, massage is uncomfortable when lying down, back massage can be carried out in a sitting or kneeling position. The best way to do this is for the woman to sit on a low stool, resting her elbows on her knees (which are apart on each side of the baby), thus giving support to the top half of her body.

With a circling stroke, use the palms of the hands to apply oil to the area to be massaged. If this is a specially sensitive area, such as the breasts or abdomen, lighten the pressure as you pass across. Talk to your partner. Ask if she prefers a firmer stroke or would like it softer. Use both hands and make circles away from the spine. This can be carried out from a straddle position across her legs but don't put much weight on her. You can also work from a kneeling position at her head – though you need to be tall in order to get a wider range of sweeping movement. Another comfortable position is for your partner to lie on her side and for you to tuck yourself close in to her thighs.

With fingertips only, lightly circle the abdomen, touching and tickling the sensitive skin. Do this over the entire abdomen for as long as you both want. It's possible for the woman to do this herself as well as having a partner do it for her. Some people find it relieves strong contractions during labour, though I didn't like to be touched this way when I was giving birth, despite having loved it during pregnancy.

This is for the back only and is a light pressure version of the glide movement used in non-pregnant massage. Place your hands, palms down at the base of the spine one on either side, fingers pointing along her body, towards her head. In the non-pregnant version you are supposed to lean the whole weight of your body on to your hands. Naturally, with a pregnant woman, this is impossible. So instead, gently push your hands up each side of her spine until they have reached her shoulders. Then bring them down the sides of her body until they meet again at the starting point.

Begin with your hands laid flat on your partner's abdomen, fingertips facing each other. Slide the hands gently past each other to the opposite side of the body, then bring them back again. Repeat this twice then move up the body a few inches and do it again. Swim up the body, lightening the stroke on the very pregnant areas and also on the breasts.

The spine is under a lot of pressure as pregnancy progresses. You can relieve this by steadying your partner with one hand on her side and rubbing gently but firmly with your other hand around the base of her spine. Occasional pressure without movement on this area is also marvellous for relaxation. Some women find the back rub invaluable during childbirth, in particular, during the type of labour known as 'back-ache' labour.

Massage strokes for mothers-to-be
CIRCLING

EFFLEURAGE

THE GLIDE

SWIMMING

THE BACK RUB

BREAST MASSAGE

This is best carried out past the three-month stage when the breasts have stopped being quite so sensitive. Kneeling at your partner's head, cup her right breast with your right hand. Slowly move your right hand gently but firmly up and over the nipple and sweep off across the top. Without letting the breast fall, instantly repeat the movement with the left hand. Continue this hand-over-hand movement for eight consecutive strokes and when the time comes to end, carefully and slowly lower her breast on to her ribcage. Repeat this hand-over-hand movement with the left breast. If it proves to be uncomfortable don't do it!

DRAINING STROKES FOR THE LEGS

The legs take a heavy pounding towards the end of pregnancy. Fluid often builds up in these areas, especially around the ankles. The pressure of the baby on blood vessels at the top of the legs and the fluid pressure also means that the circulation becomes sluggish and the legs are particularly subject to cramps.

The draining strokes used to relieve athlete's leg ache are specially useful here (see pages 102–103). Please note that if they take so long to do the partner starts needing to move, they would be best, split up into two halves. First drain the calves, second drain the thighs and, if necessary, allow time for your partner to move around in between.

PERINEAL MASSAGE

For the expectant woman to do to herself.
Gently massaging the area between vaginal entrance and anus regularly with oil may help it to become supple. In more primitive parts of the world this is regularly carried out before the birth in order to prevent unnecessary tearing during the birth.

These strokes are just a few which are adapted to suit the special conditions of pregnancy. Do remind your partner to tell what they feel like so that you can feel confident in your practice.

It is wise to be extra gentle. If you are in doubt about the suitablity of something, leave it out, especially if your partner says it is uncomfortable. If however she is irritated by your touch you are probably being too gentle and you should be firmer with the next movements. If you do accidentally hurt her, consult a doctor immediately.

Massage for the father-to-be

All the massage strokes describe in earlier chapters are suitable for expectant fathers. The only proviso is that if it is the pregnant mother who is giving the massage she only takes on movements that are easy for her to do. Anything that involves too much stretch or strain should be avoided.

Massage for mother and child

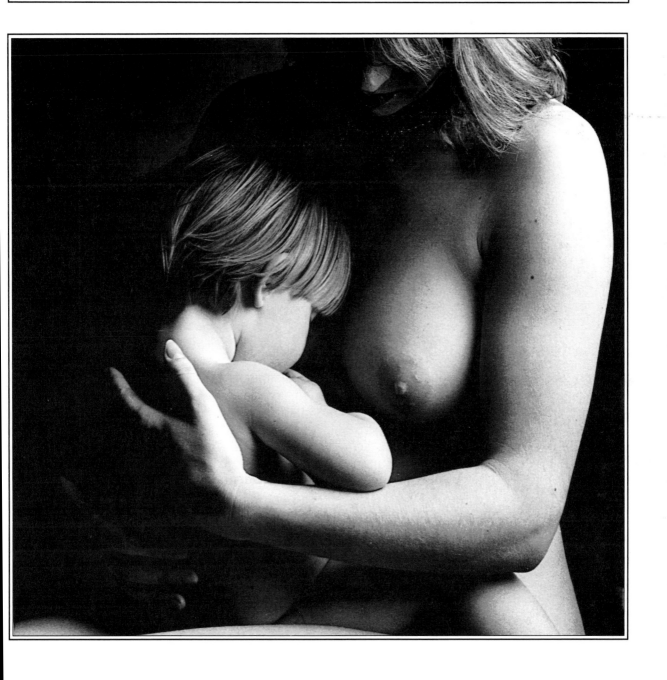

Touch is experienced by the unborn child even during the first stirrings of life. Floating securely inside the amniotic cradle it feels the viscosity of the surrounding fluid and the stroking sensations this affords when mother's sudden movement causes the baby to bob and rock. Later, during pregnancy, when the child fills the womb, its sense of enclosure is greater as it pushes and stretches against the close-fitting boundaries.

The uterus is a noisy home. Reverberating through it, pounds the deep, steady pulse of the mother's heartbeat, sudden gurgles of digestion from the stomach and any number of smaller rushing, wind sounds. These noises are both heard and *felt* by the baby since the vibrations have impact on the child's skin.

It is no coincidence therefore that enlightened obstetricians now stress the importance of reconstructing as many of these early amniotic conditions after the birth as possible, with particular emphasis on touch. Followers of the pioneering obstetricians Frederic Leboyer and Michel Odent place the newborn, slippery from birth fluids, on to the mother's stomach even before the cord is cut. Here it regains some of the warmth, comfort and body sensation of earlier days. Quiet is emphasized and wherever possible lights are dimmed. A little later (in some maternity units), the baby is bathed in body-temperature water, giving it the chance to recapture familiar floating sensations.

Touch benefits for baby

During the days that follow the birth, skin contact between mother and child is vital for the encouragement of physiological and psychological development. Animals have a habit of 'licking their newborn into shape'. Newborn bears don't look like bears until their mother have licked their flesh forcefully all over. Animals that do not receive this treatment, die.

Humans don't emulate this habit, but substitute other activities. Breast feeding, for instance, plays a vital role, not just for its nourishing qualities but also for the opportunities it affords for baby's skin to snuggle up to mother's. Rocking, hugging, patting have their function here too. One theory says that rocking tends to synchronise with the mother and baby's breathing rate, while maternal patting synchronises with the mother and baby heart rate. Breast feeding also allows the child to produce its own rocking rhythm as baby rhythmically sucks.

Rocking produces sensations which correspond to memories of amniotic floating. Rocking cradles are efficient pacifiers, as are the more fashionable rocking chairs of today. Drivers will have noted the phenomenon produced in their otherwise sleepless child where the rhythm and constant vibration of motoring sends the most colicky baby off to sleep. (My own child responds to motorway driving. Get him on the M4 and he's out like a light.)

Premature babies respond particularly well to rocking movements and touch. In one study with twins, the rocked twin gained weight at a significantly greater rate per day than the unrocked one. In another study of children with low birth-weight, the handled children were found to be more active and healthier at eight months than those who had not been handled. Premature babies regularly rocked, fondled and cuddled each day showed less likelihood of apnoea (nonbreathing) and were advanced in their central nervous system functioning. Another study comparing babies regularly touched by their mothers with babies who were not, had to be discontinued because the nurses found it too painful to watch the untouched babies without intervening.

Touch benefits for mother

The benefits of mother and baby touch aren't solely confined to the children. Clinical observation has shown that mothers who have the chance to regularly fondle their babies in the premature unit recover more rapidly themselves from pregnancy and labour than mothers whose fondling is limited.

Observations of communities where there is a 'doula' show that mothers adapt quickly to the tasks of parenthood. The doula is a motherly figure whose role is to support the new mother in the early weeks after childbirth. This takes the form of running the rest of the household, waiting on mother and child, assisting with the baby to give the mother rest and giving encouragement on an emotional level. Touch is a part of this support, with back and shoulder massage to relieve stress and breast massage to facilitate breast feeding.

Anybody can be a doula. It might be the mother's own mother, a close friend, an older woman in the community, her husband, even someone employed on a commercial basis. A doula is a caring figure who nourishes the mother's practical and emotional needs, reinforcing her abilities to parent.

Picking up sensory cues

In recent years it has become fashionable to carry baby everywhere in a sling, so that it remains in constant touch with the parent's body movement. In this way it learns about stress, taking its cues from the parent's muscular tautness in tense situations and bawling out its displeasure in spite of the mother's outwardly smiling appearance.

The plus side of this togetherness is it enables the baby to feel the mother's heartbeat and to breathe in her familiar scent and warmth-reassuring and comforting experiences. It is this ability to pick up sensory cues which may be, responsible for the difference in touch-reaction between wanted children and unwanted. One American doctor observed that mothers who did not want their children, touch more with the fingertips and this correlates with the amount of crying in their babies. In wanted pregnancy however the touch is by palm contact and the babies are calmer in the first days.

Touch benefit for father

The role of father in the early days of infancy is invaluable to mother and child, but is only just beginning to be appreciated by a society which has traditionally excluded him from the paraphenalia of babycare. He, along with his wife, possesses some of the best attributes for baby-nurture imaginable – a pair of warm hands and a loving, sensual body.

There is no iron-clad law to say that father can't carry his child in front of him in a sling, nor that his loving touch won't be just as warmly received as mother's. Far from doing this only for baby's sake, it also massively reinforces the father's own sense of self-value, not to mention creating a very important early bond between father and child.

How to massage your baby

In light of the growing research on touch for newborns, it seems extraordinary that it should still be necessary to stress its benefits. Our Western attitude to touch (it's really not quite right) stands out in massive contrast to that of the East. Russian babies, for instance, are swaddled, thus reproducing the taut conditions experienced in the womb during late pregnancy. Balinese children are always carried in a sling. Indian babies regularly receive massage from their mothers.

If there are doubts a massage might not be pleasurable, you only have to watch a baby as it is rubbed and caressed to see its pleasure. One theory about why massage may be good for a baby is that the pressure put on his or her limbs may also reproduce the taut conditions experienced by the child in the last months of pregnancy.

Massage gives a baby the opportunity to feel sensual, encourages the circulation and enhances physical and psychological development. It also allows him or her to be a warm relaxed person – attributes which he or she will be able to make good use of in later life.

Once your baby is a week old, he or she can be massaged any time, providing that the remains of the cord are avoided. However, do not massage on a full stomach or when the baby is very hungry.

Many of the adult massage strokes can be adapted for the baby, bearing in mind the recipient is tiny. It is *not* a good idea to use fast rubbing strokes, nor should you use percussion (thumping).

Be prepared for many interruptions; the baby may well want to do something else, like suckle or move, or, when it gets older, look over your shoulder. Bear them patiently but get back to the massage exercise afterwards. Slow down the strokes as you would in an adult massage, but be prepared for a baby's much shorter attention span.

The massage should be carried out in a warm room so that neither of you will feel cold at any time. Naturally your baby will be naked although it is not necessary that you are too. It is desirable to keep your legs bare since much of the massage will be performed with the baby lying there. The oil should be warmed and a box of tissues within easy reach. Sit on a large towel so that if the baby urinates which he is likely to do during the session, it won't matter. If there are other children in the room make sure there is enough space around you so that they can't trip over you.

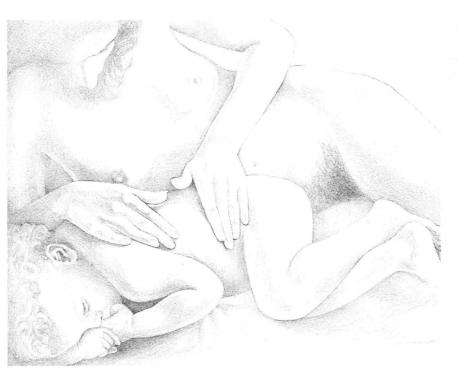

Mother and baby *Any loving touch between mother and baby will be appreciated. But be prepared for short sessions.*

It is hard to use strokes in a dramatic way on a very tiny baby since there is such a small area on which to perform. It may be necessary in such instances to use only half your hand when doing a flat hand stroke or rely on fingertip kneading.

Sitting comfortably on the floor, with your back propped up against a wall or by cushions, take the baby on your knee. Your legs should be stretched out in front of you. Coat the baby lightly with the warmed oil and then lie him on his back along your legs with his feet kicking towards your stomach.

Chest massage

With both hands laid flat on the baby's chest, move them out sideways, away from each other and down the baby's sides as if you were flattening out the baby's chest. This should be done very slowly indeed. Then return to the middle of the baby's chest and repeat the stroke a little further down. Continue with this movement until you have reached the bottom of his rib cage.

Lay both hands on the baby's shoulders and then draw them, palms down, along the baby's chest, abdomen and legs, towards you. Repeat.

A variation of this is to do the above stroke but hand over hand, first down the right side of the baby then the left, so that your hands 'swim' along.

Another variation is to glide the left hand up from the baby's left thigh across the body, ending at the right shoulder. Then follow this up immediately with the right hand, starting at baby's right thigh, pushing across the body and ending up at the left shoulder. Then repeat left and then right, so that the movement is continual.

Abdomen massage

The kneading stroke is useful here. With your fingertips pressed gently into the flesh of the baby's abdomen, slowly move the flesh in small circles, without moving the fingers on the flesh. Make these small circles all over the abdomen. This is helpful in breaking down constipation, and in moving baby's wind. Be very careful about the pressure you exert; if the baby has a sore stomach, you may hurt him. Kneading in a circle around the abdomen, following the path of the colon (clockwise) may also help.

Arms and legs massage

Turn the baby slightly on to his right side, then grasp his left hand in your left hand and, stretch out his arm. With your right hand circled around the baby's left wrist (your finger and thumb meeting together around the wrist) slowly move this bracelet-like grasp down the baby's arm until it reaches his shoulder as if your finger and thumb are 'milking' the arm.

This time hold the same hand with your *right* hand and repeat the bracelet-like milking movement using your left hand. Continue this repetitive pattern in a rhythmic movement.

As you begin each movement at the wrist, turn your hand, still in its bracelet shape, around the wrist, back and forth, back and forth, before proceeding up the arm.

When you have completed the arm strokes grasp, with both hands, around the back of the baby's hand so that your thumbs point into his palm. Then circle your thumbs on the palm in tiny circles, moving outwards from the centre of the palm towards the fingers. With a very tiny baby this may be hard to do.

Repeat this series of movements on the baby's right arm and hand.

Place the baby on his back, then repeat the sequence of movements in an identical way, to massage each of his legs in turn.

The back

Lie the baby across your knees on his stomach. Place both your hands, palms down, on the far side of his back, then slowly separate them, so that your hands are travelling away from each other, one towards his head, the other towards his feet. The hands need to start at a central point. When the far side has been 'separated' a few times, repeat on the near side.

Next, try circling with the palms of your hands in a similar manner to kneading, working your way up and down the baby's back.

Pulling the flat of your hands gently across the baby's back from the far side to the near side, one after the other, travelling up and down the back, also feels good.

Then, anchoring the baby by placing one hand on his buttocks, press lightly with the other hand on the base of the spine and glide your hand up the full length of the spine to his shoulders. Repeat a few times.

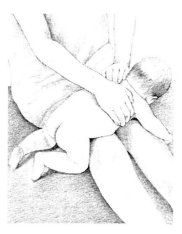

Baby back massage *Circling with the palms of your hands, work your way around your baby's back.*

Buttocks

Flat-handed massage of the baby's buttocks, mainly using the palms only, in a circular movement can be good for restoring circulation here.

Stretching

Stretch each of the baby's limbs in turn, ending with a gentle tug. Also bicycle the baby's legs, this helps to strengthen them. Gently stretching the thighs apart, then closing them together again makes the inner muscles of the thigh more supple. Carefully unfolding the child's hands helps stretch the muscles there too.

Watching babies faces while they are being massaged gives us a very clear picture of what they think: babies love massage. They stretch and gurgle in their pleasure. It feels good to know you're giving your child a rich and sensual start to life.

Skin and sex – facts and figures

* A study at the University of Colorado discovered that the parents of abused children were invariably deprived themselves of physical affection during childhood and that their adult sex life was very poor. The women never experienced orgasm and the men's sex life was unsatisfying.

* Girls have lower touch and pain thresholds than boys, a difference which remains throughout life and which shows soon after birth.

* At all ages girls are more responsive to touch than are boys.

* Girls are more dependent on sensual arousal than boys who are more dependent on visual arousal.

* Girls respond more to talking and touch than do boys. This may mean they get more of it since they will be more rewarding to pay attention to.

The young – and the old

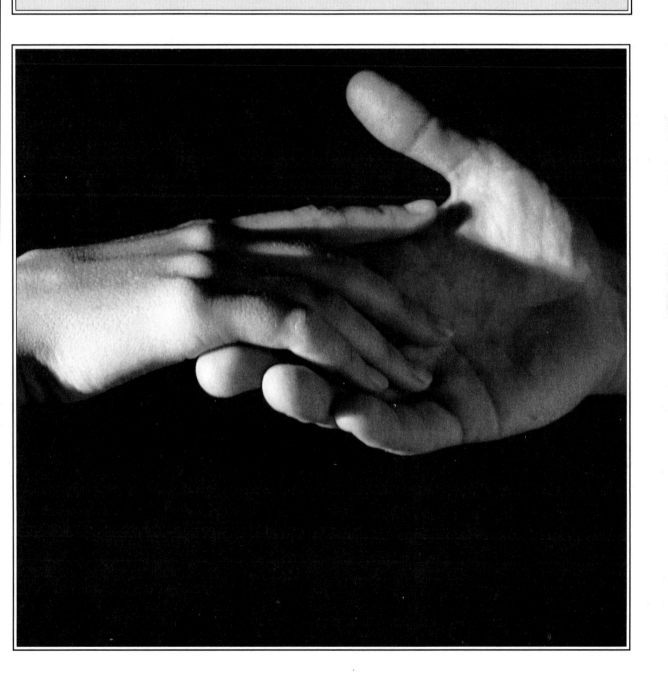

Infant touch doesn't cease when babyhood ends. Your child will grow to be a sensual toddler and will probably be rewarding his parents with big hugs and cuddles. While it's not so easy to massage a very agile toddler or pre-schooler there are other ways in which touch can be used on these older children with striking effect.

Bathtime can be great for back scrubbing and even back scratching. School age children, stiff from working at a desk, visibly relax over the tea table if you serve them up a good neck and shoulder massage. Children who are more 'sportive', may arrive home at the end of the day, with sore feet. Giving the feet a good rub with peppermint liquid soap is wonderfully refreshing. Many health shops sell Japanese foot rollers. These are small, turned, wooden cylinders that roll beneath your feet, pressing on the nerves and pressure points in the soles. The most minor claim for foot rolling is that it feels lovely. The most extravagant claim comes from one man who couldn't keep up with his much older father on hikes because his father possessed an infinitely greater store of energy. This was the result, the claim went, of rolling his feet on a wooden roller, every day of his life. School children, constantly pounding the playground and playing-field, find roller massage invigorating too.

Touch games can add a lot of fun to children's parties. I dimly remember one party when I was eight years old, where I was blindfolded and taken on a touch tour of my friends home, a grisly tale recounted as we went. The two things that really stick in my mind were being forced to hold 'a convicts' eyeballs that had been 'wrenched from his head'. I was given two round, wet objects which felt exactly like eyes. With a scream I ripped the blindfold off and saw that I was actually holding a pair of peeled grapes.

A little later in the game I was told (blindfolded again) that as a punishment I had to sniff and then drink the same unfortunate's 'urine'. I was given an evil smelling liquid I was forced to down. Almost vomiting, I was convinced it *was* urine but, amidst roars of laughter, my friends assured me it was really dandelion wine! Ugh!

Years later I was reminded of this childhood game again when an enterprising theatre group turned a glamorous version of it into a theatrical experience, and surfeited the audience every night by leading them blindfold through rooms of velvet and silk, feeding them with exotic fruit, stroking them with peacock feathers and playing sweet music. All the senses were pampered.

Teenagers, as noted at the beginning of this book, withdraw from parental touch when they begin to be sexually aware. The bathroom door is all of a sudden locked and it becomes important that young people are allowed privacy. A massage will *not* be welcomed at this stage in life – unless it is for something specific. It is perfectly acceptable to have sun tan oil applied while on the beach, in a 'creative' manner. A spot massage is usually acceptable to an aching teenage back after a hard game of tennis.

The fact that teenagers withdraw though is no excuse to let them go short on family hugs. If your children are used to being hugged, they'll miss it if you suddenly stop. If you are used to tucking their arm in under yours when shopping, carry right on doing it. If they don't like it they will remove their body from your immediate vicinity. But experience with my own teenage sons has taught me that they like the occasional chance of being close to their parents, even if they don't want it prolonged. The touch however needs to be on non-sexual areas. Remembering my increasing annoyance at my father's habit of patting me on the bottom as a teenager (something he'd done for years previously without me giving a thought to it) I wouldn't do it to a teenager myself.

Grans and grandpas are people who respond to a good cuddle too. One of the conundrums of age is that although the skin loses its elasticity and some of its ability to feel, age seems to bring on a greater urge to be touched. We have an unfeeling attitude (I use the adjective deliberately) to old people and the clear signs of touch starvation amidst the elderly probably derive from the simple fact they don't get very much of it.

Loss of a lifetime partner hits us all eventually and one of the least-discussed aspects of the loss is the deprivation of human touch. The warmth, comfort and cuddling that goes on between two people with a happy relationship disappears at a stroke. The shock to the one left behind is great.

It's this loss of tactile connection which is responsible for so many old ladies keeping cats. Cats are sleek and sensual creatures, rewarding to pet and warm to hold. Another attempt to compensate for touch starvation explains the large numbers of older women who become passionate about reflexology in their later years. Reflexology teaches you massage skills which concentrate on certain key spots in the hands and feet. By stimulating these spots, you also, it is claimed, stimulate a variety of glands in the body. Some people think that this rejuvenates. What is important about reflexology however is that you are given a legitimate method of *touching yourself*. It may not be the same as cuddling with a lover but it is a great improvement on the lonely alternative of no touch at all.

I am drawn back time and again to the description Kate the social worker gave me of using massage with the old people who were in her care (p. 41). Their gratitude for being given Kate's touch was so moving that Kate had tears in her eyes when she told me the story. There's a moral to be learned here. Whenever possible, go out and massage a granny or a grandpa today. They will love it!

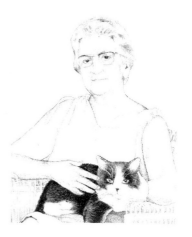

The warmth and companionship of a cat can help compensate for the loss of a lifetime partner.

Massage for old people

All the massages recommended for young or middle-aged people are appropriate for older men and women provided adequate massage oil is used. Older skin is usually dryer and possesses less elasticity but carefully manipulated brings much pleasure to its possessor.

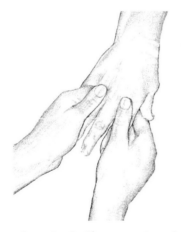

Take great care to be gentle with old people. Do not tug at the hair in a head massage.

The main safeguard to practise is to keep a careful watch for reddening of the skin, a sign that pressure is being over done. If you have fears that your touch is too firm for an old person ask them how it feels. It may be wise to avoid head and hair manipulation since loss of hair is a problem of old age and no one wants to feel responsible for accelerating it. Similarly heavy pressure strokes on bones (such as the glide) should be left out.

The anti-stress massages (outlined on pages 103–106) for the head are good for older people. The only alteration to make here is in the *forehead* and *temple* press. Make these extra gentle.

Most of the *facial strokes* in this section are excellent for old people because they are all gentle ones. The neck and shoulder rubs may prove wonderful for relieving stress but take care to find out if the man or woman sufferers from any arthritic or rheumatic condition. If this is the case neck massage is best left to the professionals.

Hand and *foot* massages are specially acceptable to older men and women. For foot massage see page 17. For hand massage see below.

Hand massage

Thumb circling Knead gently between the bones on the back of the hand. Watch carefully for any sign of reddening of the skin indicating too firm pressure is being applied.

Thumb circling the back of the hand. Holding one of your partners hands, back uppermost in both of yours, grasp with the four fingers of each of your hands and use your thumbs. First, slowly push both thumbs simultaneously along the grooves made between the bones on the back of the hand. Repeat until all grooves have been kneaded gently upwards.

Hand bending. Holding their wrist with one hand, carefully and slowly bend their hand backwards by pushing your fingertips against theirs. Stop when it will bend no further. But repeat a couple of times.

Hand flexing. Holding your partner's arm by the elbow to steady it, hold their fingers in your other hand. Slowly rotate the hand so that it is turning at the wrist.

Finger massage. Taking each of your partner's fingers in turn (including the thumbs) hold them at the base between your fingers and thumb and work your way in a kneading fashion upwards and off at the end. Repeat this movement two or three times with each finger finishing by gently pulling the finger away from the socket then letting go.

Between the fingers. Run one of your fingers, preferably the forefinger, backwards and forwards between each of theirs at the base, next to the hand, several times. This gives a very sensual sensation.

Palm pressing with the thumbs. Hold the hand firmly with both of your own, your fingers at the back and your thumbs resting on their palms. Firmly press for several seconds with your thumbs on to the fleshy parts of their hand, then rest. Repeat until all fleshy areas have been covered.

Thumb kneading. Holding the hand as before, knead the fleshy parts of their palm with our thumbs working towards their thumb. As you reach it alter your strokes so that you pull away up the thumb as you did in the finger massage stroke.

Thumb pulling. Holding their hand underneath with their palm uppermost, pull the ball of your thumb hard across the fleshy ridge on your partner's palm immediately below their fingers. Repeat the movement slowly several times. Some people like this movement enlarged to circle right around the palm, keeping the fleshy areas on the outside of it.

Hand to hand palming. Holding their hand from underneath as before but placing it actually on your knee or their knee if that is most comfortable, place the palm of your other hand over their palm with the heel of your hand fitting into the centre of theirs. With quite a deep pressure rotate their hand with the heel of yours. It may also prove necessary to stabilise their hand with the fingers of your hand that is doing the rotating.

Whole hand rotation. Grasp their hand (back uppermost) with both yours at each side and stretch out their arm. Then gently tilt your hands from side to side in small rotating circles in a continual movement.

When one hand has been completed, repeat the sequence on the other.

Many of these strokes can be done by an older person to themself and a further study of reflexology movements for the hands may also be of use.

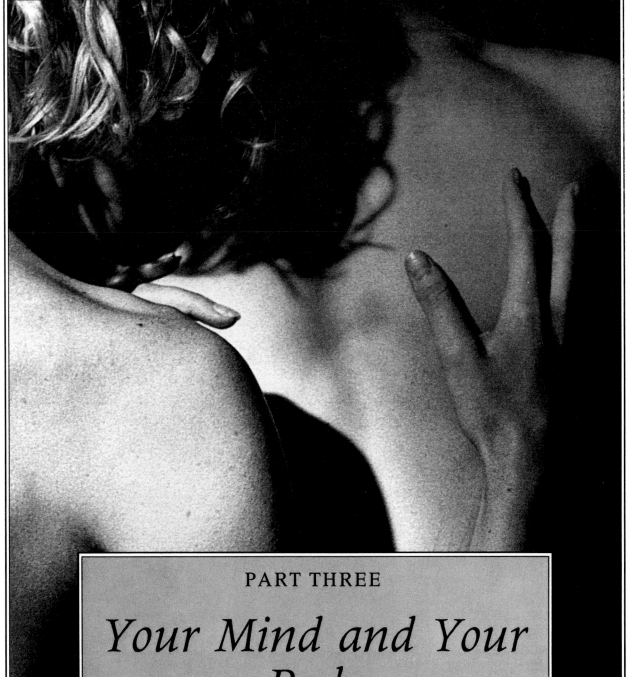

PART THREE

Your Mind and Your Body

Keeping fit

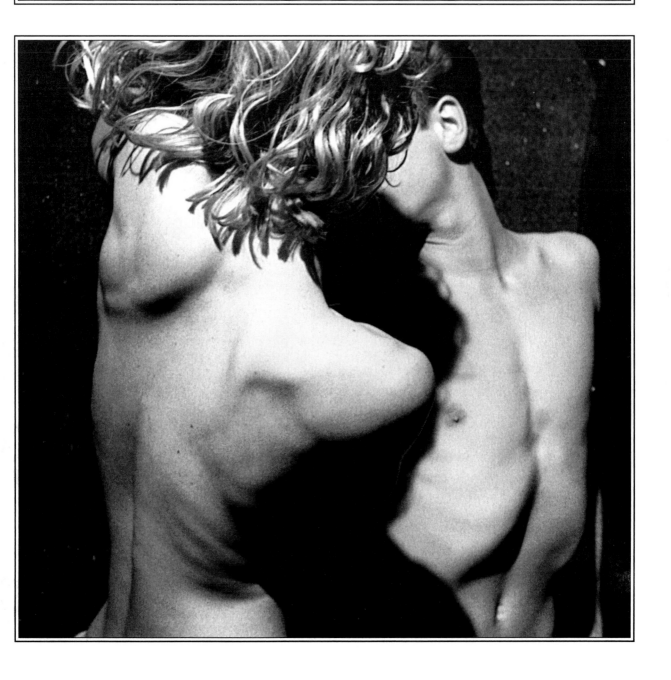

Extensive research has shown that a combination of exercise and careful diet are the best ingredients for fitness. What has been omitted from the majority of health information to date is the fact that touch, and in particular, massage, can help make you fit too.

When we jog, the movement of our body pumps extra oxygen around our veins, enabling fat to be burned up. Massage is a 'lazy' way of facilitating exactly this process. Instead of moving our body with our own muscles, the masseur's hands 'make the running'.

Massage increases blood flow and simultaneously increases oxygen circulation. The extra oxygen is then used by the metabolic system to burn up fat deposits. But massage *alone* will *not* make you miraculously fit or lose weight. If it did, sport would be redundant and diet-inventors bankrupted years ago. What it does do is accelerate a fitness programme if used in association with exercise and diet.

How massage can help

Together with diet

Massage can be used to improve digestion. Spot massaging, that is working specifically on offending areas (commonly thighs and buttocks), localises the increased fat 'burn-up'. It actually changes the shape of your body by breaking down fat cells under the skin already reduced by dieting (see page 101).

Colonic massage (see page 48) aids peristalsis by breaking down waste matter in the colon, thus allowing it to move more efficiently to the bowel. The more thoroughly we are able to expel food waste the less weight we retain.

As more is discovered about the causes of obesity we are learning that a person's mental attitude towards their body can affect their weight. The eating groups, founded by the women's health movement, have demonstrated that the ability to eat carefully grows spontaneously when an obese person accepts and feels happy about their appearance. One of the spin-offs of massage, particularly when used within a therapeutic group, is helping people come to terms with their appearance. Group massage sessions have lifted depressions, enabling such problems as overweight and skin blemishes to miraculously disappear. One theory about weight loss is that the removal of stress, which massage facilitates, allows the digestive system to function more efficiently, with the welcome side-effect of cheering you up!

Together with exercise

When people begin to jog they usually feel some pain as a result of the unaccustomed exercise. This is caused by the build-up of acidic wastes which are drawn out by fatigue. The removal of these wastes is speeded up by an accelerated blood flow, which massage encourages. Once the pain disappears, a sense of achievement and pleasure takes it place; the athlete begins to enjoy the sport. Specific massage draining techniques are of special value here (see page 102–103).

However, note that although some people think that massaging an injury is the best way to accelerate healing, this is a myth. Massage aggravates the wound. It not only increases internal bleeding but, on a severe injury, might stimulate blood clotting and bone formation in torn muscle fibres. The only touch which should be ventured is the light smoothing of an anti-coagulant cream (heparinoid) or arnica cream on the bruised area.

Skin disorders

Touch has a special relationship to skin disorders. In past centuries the common people believed their king or queen possessed the power to heal by touch. They would present themselves at regular touch sessions in order to try and clear their skins. Since some of the conditions did improve there seemed grounds for believing that the method worked. However, when analysed in 1825, the royal touch was found to have worked with only a tiny percentage of sufferers. Present perspective of such healing might classify this as faith healing rather than touch therapy.

However, medical opinion today says that there *is* a value in the power of touch for people with skin problems and that it is impossible to separate the mind from the body in this instance, since one works in conjunction with the other. Eczema is a condition to which this view applies.

One thesis maintains that certain children may be predisposed to eczema because they didn't obtain adequate soothing from their mothers. Dr Maurice J Rosenthal tested this by surveying twenty-five mothers with children under the age of two who were suffering from eczema and the majority of them did indeed fail to give the children much comforting touch.

Psychoanalysis recognises that in frustrating situations, symptoms, of anger are sometimes expressed as itching and scratching. Subsequent psychotheraphy on the powerful underlying emotions often has the side-effect of clearing up the pruritus.

Self-esteem can be a powerful healer for people with skin disorders too. The discovery that others feel perfectly happy about touching skin that the sufferer feels to be disfigured can so alter the sufferer's self-esteem that both spots and depression melt away.

The power of touch

Touch is used therapeutically by physiotherapists, osteopaths and chiropractors in a range of specialised movements. Muscles which come under stress, as a result of say a bone condition, can be aided by special massage. The pain is eased even if the bone condition is not cured.

Touch was observed by Professor of Psychiatry, James Lynch, of the University of Maryland School of Medicine in Baltimore to protect animals from feeling pain. In experiments with dogs and horses he discovered that whereas under normal conditions they showed a drastic increase in heart rate if given an electric shock on the leg, when the same animals were petted while being given the shock, their heart-beat remained normal. Some of the animals did not even flex their legs in reaction to the pain. As a result of these observations Professor Lynch and his colleagues turned their attention towards humans. They observed patients whose hearts were constantly monitored in intensive care units. They found significant changes in heart rate and rhythm from such simple contact as the nurse routinely taking the patient's pulse. Even if the patient was in a coma, the heart responded markedly to touch.

Dolores Krieger is a professor of nursing at New York University who has become famous for her study and development of the 'healing touch' – a modern version of the laying on of hands. One of her students, Patricia Heidt, measured the anxiety levels of hospital patients admitted with suspected heart attacks before and after three types of five-minute 'treatments'. In one situation, a nurse talked to the patient for five minutes without touching. This usually sent the patient's anxiety level soaring. In another 'treatment' the nurse offered five minutes of 'therapeutic touch'. She told the patient, 'I'm going to use my hands in a way I've been taught, to try and help you' and concentrated on sending healing energies, holding her hands a few inches above the patient's skin. Despite the strangeness of this activity, patients showed a significant reduction in anxiety. The third 'treatment' consisted of taking the patient's pulse in four different places over five minutes. This also significantly reduced anxiety levels.

Professor Krieger breaks down the therapeutic touch into several constituents. The first consists of *centering*. As in yoga, the healer needs to relax, to turn inwards mentally and to clear the mind. Secondly, the healer extends the hands so that they hover about two or three inches above the area where the discomfort is sited. Having done this they 'tune in' to the layers of 'heat' that they sense between themselves and the sufferer. At this stage they do what is called an *assessment*, feeling in their own hand, degrees of heat, cold, prickles and so on which indicate disruption in the sufferer's energy. Thirdly the healer, by the power of thought directed through the hands, balances the sufferer's disrupted energies. This is described as *'unruffling'*, changing the heat, cold, prickles to the normal warmth that the energy field is supposed to consist of. Fourthly, comes the *withdrawal* stage when the healer recognises it is time to stop and withdraws the hands.

In her book *The Therapeutic Touch* Professor Krieger details a number of exercises to test whether or not you are approaching a suitable level of consciousness for healing. These include practising on a friend, becoming aware of feeling in your own hands, and practising on animals such as the pet cat to 'tune in' to their energy field. One of the theories behind this is that every living creature possesses its own field of energy (possibly a form of electricity) – a theory supported by Kirlian photography (which demonstrates by photograph that every living thing possesses a type of 'electric' force field). On this basis the healer is intervening in the individual's energy field, by the use of psychokinetic power, in order to re-arrange it. Both Russian and American tests have shown it is possible to move *objects* by psychokinetic power. Perhaps it is possible to move energy fields too.

Whether or not you believe this, the fact remains that massage, the actual laying on of hands, *can* wipe out a headache without drugs, *can* relieve stress symptoms so that the sufferer calms down and *can* dispel muscular aches and pains.

Touch can also enhance people's feelings and memories. Studies show that if shop assistants touch people when they hand out change, they are more likely to be remembered than if they don't. Similarly, in a public library, the librarian who touches you while handling your books is more likely to be recalled than the librarian who doesn't.

On this basis touch can be used to help promote a career if managed thoughtfully. Shaking hands firmly at a job interview has, for years, been recommended as a way of creating a good impression. Seniors, in an office, who touch juniors on the shoulder occasionally, are regarded with warmth, although this doesn't work the other way round. The junior who is too 'touchy' with a senior would be regarded as pushy and attention seeking, and the senior who overdoes the touching would probably be penalised by his union for sexual harassment! Nevertheless there is a place for shaking hands at meetings and farewells which, although old-fashioned, builds up esteem for the instigator.

Massaging for health

THE BUTTOCK SQUASH

Running up and down stairs regularly is one of the best exercises to help get rid of a pear-shaped derrière. But kneading and 'squashing' the bottom every day over a period of six to eight weeks can also help strengthen this area and bring back suppleness. Kneading usually consists of grasping large folds of flesh and rolling it between thumb and finger tips as you would a piece of dough.

Using the kneading stroke with both hands, work firmly up and down your partner's buttocks in long sweeps of movement. Then work from side to side across your partner's bottom taking care to miss out the bony end of the spine.

The same kneading stroke can be used for *spot massage* on areas of extra fat.

FINGERTIP HACKING

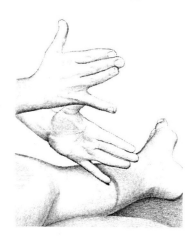

Percussion movements such as hacking and clapping, don't have to be so powerful that they hurt the person being massaged. Their aim should be to provide enough vibration to stimulate the tissues immediately below the surface of the skin. Hacking consists of hitting the partner's skin with the edge of your hands and little fingers, first one hand, then the other, in a barrage of light blows. The movement is taken from the wrist so there is no destructive power behind it but is rather like the light wrist movement used in drum practice! These strokes are good for the sides of the buttocks (from just below the hip) and on the fatty parts of the thighs.

CLAPPING

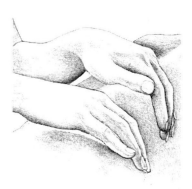

Clapping is another simple percussion movement, where, keeping your thumbs close in to your fingers, you clap your partner's body with first one hand, then the other, continuously, and near enough to each other so that one thumb is brushing the other. This can be used on almost every part of the body, but is most effective on areas like the thighs and the calves.

Aiding weight loss
COLONIC MASSAGE

This series of on-the-spot rotations, following the line of the colon, helps loosen up and expel waste matter (see page 48).

Sporting aids
DRAINING MASSAGE

This massage can be used after intense exercise to aid the release of painful acidic waste from the muscles. *Sequence one* consists of squeezing the lower leg with both hands pressed around your partner's ankle and slowly but firmly pressing your hands, like a large bracelet, up your partner's leg towards the knee. As you progress a roll of flesh should appear in front of your index fingers and visually it looks as if you are pushing this roll of flesh right the way up the leg. You are not, of course, but you are emptying the veins in the lower leg for a few moments, aiding the action of the blood towards the heart and draining the area of the acidic waste gathered there.

Sequence two can be carried out on the thigh. First prepare the thigh with kneading and clapping strokes (see pages 101 and 102). Then move down the leg to the foot. Cup both your hands around your partner's ankle with the whole of each hand touching the partner's skin. Your hands should be positioned one above the other, with fingers pointing in opposite directions. Press your hands all the way to the top of the legs, only lightening pressure over the knees. On the thigh you may see a similar roll of flesh appear in front of your leading hand. When you reach the top of the thigh, turn the hands, circling out and down, making just light contact with the side of the leg. Then resume the position at the ankle and start again. Repeat this sequence ten times in a flowing series of unbroken movements. This series of rhythmic sweeps aids the flow of blood towards the heart.

Preceding these strokes with kneading is *vital* as preparation for the draining.

Sequence Three treats the arms in a similar fashion. This massage should be preceded by careful thumb kneading strokes over the upper arms up on to the shoulders and around the thickly muscled parts between shoulder and elbow, several times. When you come to draining the arm, it is best to prop the arm up so that your partner's hand is resting on your shoulder, where you can hold it in place by trapping it with your head, squeezing it against your shoulder. The draining then goes from wrist to elbow, skirts lightly over the elbow and continues up to the shoulder.

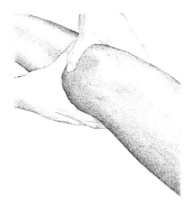

Draining *Squeeze your partner's leg with both hands at the ankle and slowly press the hand, like a large bracelet, up towards the knee.*

The two places where stress most commonly shows up in the human body are in the head (headaches) and in the spine (neck ache and back ache). The following strokes are specifically suggested to smooth away pain from these areas.

Anti-stress massage

Find out exactly where the headache is experienced. Both first and last movements in a headache massage should consist of direct pressure for a few seconds on this spot.

MASSAGING AWAY A HEADACHE

Begin with a *forehead press*. Lay one hand across the forehead, then the other hand on top of the first. Contact must be even from all parts of your lower hand. Gently lean on the forehead for a count of thirty, then relax.

Temple press – don't lift your hands off but rather separate them out so that they are now each making contact with the forehead, one on either side of the temples. If your hands are too large to fit comfortably (palms should be on the temples, fingers on the forehead), swivel the fingers upwards into the hairline, allowing the rest of the hands to have better contact. Hold the hands lightly in place for a few seconds and then give a light press for a few seconds. Then relax for another couple of seconds before lifting off.

Stroking the forehead – cover the forehead with one hand as in the forehead press, then sweep that hand down, as far as the bridge of the nose, before lifting off. Before you lift off begin the same movement with the other hand down towards the nose. This is a hand-over-hand sequence. Repeat ten times.

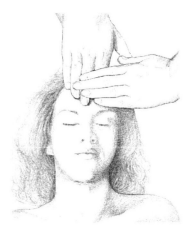

Fingertip pressure *Press down on the forehead with fingertips from one hand reinforced by the fingertips from the other at right angles*

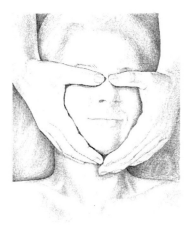

Eye pressure *Rest the ball of the thumb lightly on the eyelid for a count of 20, then lift or gently sweep off, across the eye.*

Fingertip pressure – press down on the forehead for a count of thirty with four fingertips from the left hand, reinforced by four fingers from the right hand positioned directly on top. Relax the pressure. Shift the top hand to a right angle over the bottom one and use it to press down the lower fingers once again for a count of thirty. Weave the top fingers in between the bottom fingers so that now eight fingertips are pressing down for a count of thirty. Complete the sequence with the forehead press.

Forehead circling – if the headache persists, press down with four fingertips from one hand on to the forehead. Keeping the fingers in one place on the skin, move the skin itself in tiny circles. Circle all over one side of the forehead then switch to the other hand and circle the other side. The fingertips can be used, similarly, *without* much pressure, on the temples.

Eye pressure – with both hands cupped around the partner's cheeks position the thumbs above the eyes and rest the ball of the thumb lightly on the eyelid for a count of twenty then lift off. Rest the ball of the thumb once more on the eyes and very gently sweep across the eyes, moving from the inside corner of the eye to the outer corner of the eye where you sweep off.

Circling the eye – holding down the forehead with one hand, make contact with your partner's eyelid with a single finger. Very lightly and very gently circle around the surface of the eyelid. Repeat on the other eye.

Eye socket stroking – hold the centre of the forehead down with both your thumbs and place the tips of each little finger in the inside corner of each eye. Press down gently then pull the finger across the top of the eye, pressing half against the eye and half into the socket. While this fingertip is moving towards the outside corner (with gentle pressure), repeat the process with the next finger (the third) so that it is following the little one. Then the second finger and finally the first, so that all four, one by one, have taken it in turn to follow the other to the outside corner. Once all four fingers have travelled across, make a couple of light circling strokes with the four fingertips held together on the temples before returning them to starting position. Throughout this movement the thumbs continue to act as anchors at the centre of the forehead. Then repeat. The same movement can also be carried out on the lower eye socket below the eye. Your fingertips are travelling between the eye and the socket in this movement.

Complete the headache massage with a final forehead press on the area which was originally painful.

This collection of strokes works like magic with stress headaches and tension. The heaviest day in the office can be endured with the knowledge that ten to fifteen minutes of this will transform you.

NECK STRAIN   Since the neck has to support that heavy load – the head – it's one of the prime targets for pain. One way of relieving neck ache is to use kneading strokes on the painful area. Both thumb kneading and fingertip kneading, starting from one side of the shoulders, working right up into the neck and then travelling on to the other side of the shoulders, relaxes the muscles there, smoothing the pain away.

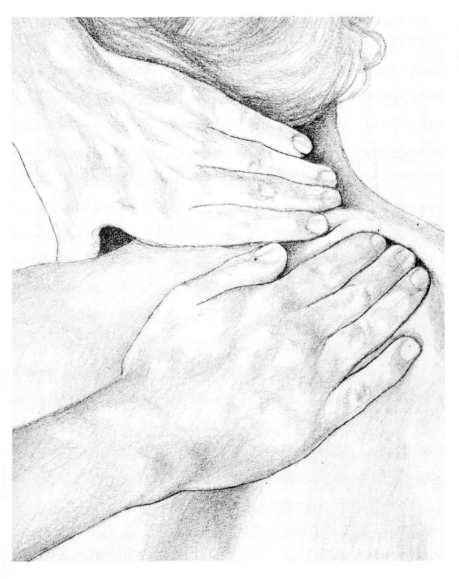

Neck Strain *Relax the muscles and soothe away pain using firm fingertip kneading from one side of the shoulders up the neck, moving on to the other side of the shoulders.*

BACK ACHE

The lower part of the spine takes the main strain of holding the body upright. Small wonder that it sometimes complains. Heavy people are specially prone to back ache. There are two strokes which are wonderful for relaxing this area.

Hand press – your partner lies on their stomach and you are positioned across their legs. Place your hands, palms down, on each side of the spine (not on the spine itself) at the waist. Then lean forward on to your hands and let the weight of your body naturally part your hands as they slip over to the side and off your partner's body. Then repeat the movement a little further down the back, until you reach the top of the buttocks. The pressure of your hands, smoothes the aches away, out of the spine and the sides of the body.

If this doesn't quite do the trick, there is probably some *thumb kneading* to be done on the areas of skin at the side of the spine just below the ribs, progressing down to the buttocks. Sometimes you can actually feel the knotted muscles below the surface, but you can also feel them relax as a result of your kneading.

Touch for a better world

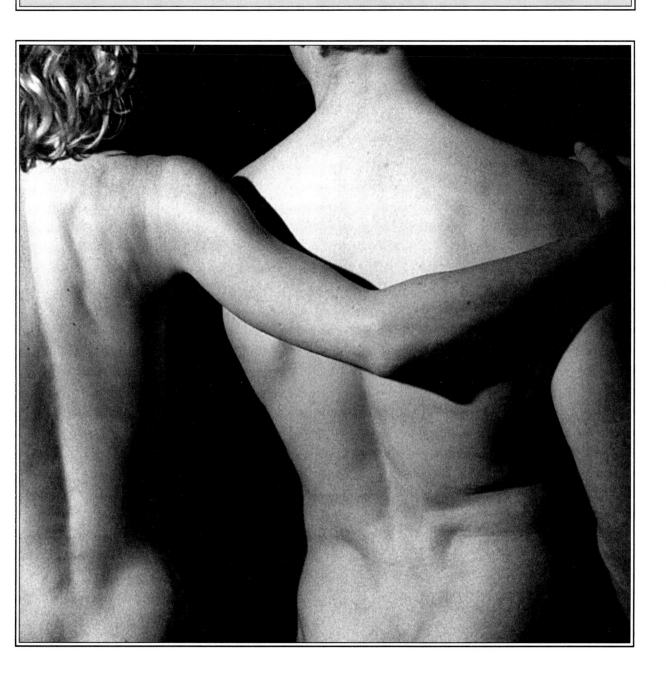

If it were compulsory that *everyone* were massaged for one hour, once a day, world wars might be a thing of the past, and aggression and tension a dim primeval memory. Brain experiments have shown that pain cannot be experienced at the same time as pleasure and that the more pleasure recipients get the more they want. Admittedly this work was carried out on animals, but there is every reason to think that humans share these propensities.

Ideally, if children are touched and caressed during infancy, they will grow up to be caring, peace-loving individuals. It is when this touch ceases and our bodies are starved that detrimental physical change occurs. If we continued touch throughout adulthood we could love rather than hate, make peace not war, and care about *each other* because we, ourselves, were happy.

Compulsory massage is of course partly a joke and partly an eccentric point of view, but there's the germ of an idea in it. Science fiction writers have already created utopias around the idea of free touch, although this is usually confused with free sex. I, in a fantasy feature for *Cosmopolitan* magazine, once advanced the proposition that all violent criminals should be punished with compulsory loving – this consisting of daily demonstrations of love such as massage, hugging, stroking and nurturing. Battering mothers would be taken away from their children and put through intensive courses of being loved until they were deemed capable of being loving themselves and then allowed to rejoin their baby.

Of course with this kind of fantasy punishment on the statute books it would be reasonable to expect over-full prisons for a while, but since, in my utopia, everyone would be able to receive as much touching and nurture as they wanted (as well as their regular daily dose), it would rapidly become unnecessary to punish people at all.

My fantasy ideas were based on touch for rehabilitation work that had already been tested and found to work. If we can see that rigorous touch can help autistic and brain-damaged children, wreak miracles with schizophrenics and allow socially maladjusted teenagers to re–adjust, it ought to follow logically that if we all had adequate amounts of touching, the world would become a happier place.

It wouldn't, of course, prevent famine, natural disaster and over-population. But it might result in an even sharing of resources across the planet so that the African millions, for instance, don't starve, while the richer Americans adjust to a diet of lentils and brown rice (not such a bad thing).

Of course, there are many reasons why such a system *wouldn't* work. One such is that there are anomalies in our chromosome make-up which decree that some people are genetically programmed to become more aggressive than others. Yet in a world where the majority of humans felt well-disposed towards each other, perhaps even hormonal aggression could be overcome. Experts might find a way to develop hormone replacement which dissipated aggression and allowed the violent to lead less disturbed lives.

It is not such an extravagant claim to state that if, nation wide, people felt happier, more relaxed, less depressed, less tired and fitter, they would also be in a frame of mind to help people rather than create difficulties for themselves. Touch, to my mind, is a simple human resource, which is capable of doing this. It costs nothing except time.

A couple of years ago, some English students delegated one of the summer months as a 'touch month'. They encouraged everyone to touch someone warmly at least once a day during this period. The feedback they received was deeply encouraging. The 'touchers' experienced a sense of fun and friendship which wasn't normally present in their lives. We can learn from this experiment. Massage someone today!

Reading list

Touch by Ashley Montague (Harper, Colophon Books).   **Touch**

The Art of Sensual Massage by Gordon Inkeles and Murray Todris   **Massage**
(Unwin Paperbacks).
The Massage Book by George Downing (Penguin).
Massage and Peaceful Pregnancy by Gordon Inkeles (Unwin Paperbacks).
The New Massage by Gordon Inkeles (Unwin Paperbacks).

The Therapeutic Touch by Dolores Krieger (Spectrum).   **Health**

The Body Electric by Anne Hooper (Unwin Paperbacks).   **Sex therapy**
The Thinking Woman's Guide to Sex by Anne Hooper (Futura).
Treat Yourself to Sex by Paul Brown and Carolyn Faulder (Penguin).
Understanding Human Sexual Inadequacy by Belliveau & Richter
(Coronet).

Index

A

B